How To Heal Scar Tissue

Work With Your Own Scar Tissue to Get Rid of It!

by Jonathan Kraft, CMT

- The Legal Schtuff -

By reading this book, I agree that I understand the following:

A massage therapist is not a medical doctor, and does not treat or diagnose medical conditions. Nor does a massage therapist prescribe medications, or therapies in a medical realm. I understand that individuals' experiences from reading this book are just their experiences, and that my results may vary from theirs.

Further, I agree to hold harmless and not liable, anyone involved in the writing or production of this book, for any results I may or may not have. (Although, when I have great results from practicing what is offered here, I will try to remember to write a nice thank-you note to the author.)

My continued reading of this book says that I agree to all of the above.

Oh, and I also agree that if I choose to act like a monkey, people might treat me like one.

So basically, by reading this book, you're agreeing that you are taking what I offer you as simple advice from a friend who wants to help. You agree that you won't sue me for taking my experiences and sharing them with you.

How To Heal Scar Tissue -
Hey, Don't Touch Me!
How to Work With Your Own Scar Tissue to Get Rid of It!
by Jonathan Kraft

A lot of times, when a person has had a surgery or an accident, which results in scar tissue formation, he or she subconsciously view the area as broken or ugly. Because of society's standards of what is pretty and what is ugly, a lot of times, the scar tissue that forms, is, by many people's standards, ugly.

Scar tissue can also be painful, seem unnatural, and feel uncomfortable. These feelings about scar tissue often lead people to subconsciously and consciously ignore an area which has scar tissue built up in it, and can lead to them feeling like they don't ever want to be touched in that area again.

This is especially true when the scarring occurs in parts of the body that someone feels uncomfortable with before the scar tissue forms. That is why this book is called, *Hey, Don't Touch Me! How to Work With Your Own Scar Tissue to Get Rid of It!* I am going to give you specific ways to work through the scar tissue in your body.

See this monkey?

The monkey represents you, the reader.

Yes, dear reader, I realize that it's not a very flattering picture, but it's the most recent one that was available.

I hope you will forgive me. I really wish that this book was interactive and that you could actually ask me questions as you are reading it, but in absence of that, I am going to try to be you, reading this book for the first time, and ask questions for you as we go through the book.

SO WHY DID YOU CHOOSE THIS MONKEY TO REPRESENT **ME**? I JUST **BOUGHT YOUR BOOK** AND NOW I'M A MONKEY???

Whoa! You don't have to get so angry. Besides, you're kind of cute, don't you think?

There are reasons that this picture was chosen to represent you. It represents the way a lot of people feel about their scar tissue.

Notice a few things about this monkey (i.e. you)
1. The stern look, and beady eyes, saying "Behind this mean face, all I really want is someone to take care of me, hug me, tell me everything will be okay, and that things will be better soon."
2. The flaring nostrils, showing everyone "I'm especially frustrated that I can't move a specific part of my body very well."
3. The bared teeth, implying "If you come any closer to my scar, I will eat you."

The book is divided into three parts, and is really designed to help you (you cute little monkey you!) through a humorous approach (after all, laughter is the best medicine), to work through the scar tissue formations in your body.

In other words, consider this the table of contents.

Part I. "Hey, How DID This Happen?"   6
Why do I have scar tissue?

This book starts with the basics:
- What is scar tissue?   17
    - Body responses
    - Time for creation!
    - Why is it so lumpy?

- Why does scar tissue form?
    - Ouch! That hurts!   20
    - Physiology and Psychology
    - It's not just in my head!

Part II. "Hey, I Need to Know!"   24
Can this really work? And how can I massage or work with my scar tissue As the book progresses, it becomes more specific. Part II gives ways to massage scar tissue in a general sense. There is then a section on how to massage scar tissue in each of the following areas:

- Knees   34
- Elbows   41
- Face   45
- Abdominals   49
- Uterine   53
- Breasts   58
- Back   61
- Shoulders   67
- Feet   71
- other parts and considerations   76

Part III. "Hey, I'm busy!"   78
How can I do this in my crazy schedule?

Part of the problem that people often face when trying to improve their health and well-being, not just when it comes to scar tissue, but health in general, is that it takes more time to stretch, massage, and eat healthfully. People often don't make changes to improve their health due to the various time constraints of their life.

Part III deals with the time it takes to heal your body. Time is a valuable commodity which we all seem to have less and less of these days. So the book concludes with ways that you can incorporate massage and stretching into your daily routines. It gives you practical ways to apply some of the techniques explained in Part II, without taking time away from what you currently do. This gives you ways to heal your scar tissue in the midst of doing the things you already do.

There is a real need for people to take their own healing on themselves, as a lot of what is currently being done in Western medicine encourages people to just pop a pill and try to work through, or completely ignore, the pain. The goals of the exercises and instructions in the book are to help you increase your range of motion, increase circulation, increase flexibility, and decrease pain. My goal is, through this book, to help you live a happier life, by giving you back the physical mobility you once had.

Scar tissue healing takes time, but through deciding to work on your healing (which is probably what brought you to this book), you can learn to work through your scar tissue and live a happier and more fulfilling life.

PART I. Hey! How DID this happen?
Why do I have Scar Tissue?

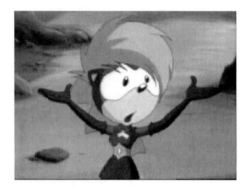

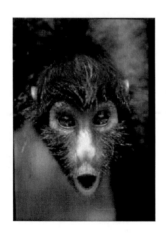

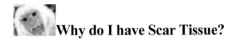Why do I have Scar Tissue?

Hopefully you won't find this part of the book too boring. But if you do think it's boring, well, just skip it!

No... don't do that... keep reading. I really will try to keep it from getting dry or thick, or scientific, although we will be looking at a lot of scientific concepts which you should have at least a basic understanding of, before diving into your healing process.

(And I've thrown in my comments along the way, so hopefully you will enjoy reading the "science-ish" stuff a bit more if that's not your cup of tea.)

BODY RESPONSES

Scar tissue is a body response. If we are active and healthy, we contribute to the breakdown and regeneration of our bodies through our daily activities. The body is constantly in a breaking down/rebuilding process. Skin on the epidermis layer, which is the outermost layer of the skin regenerates itself approximately every 28 days, and regeneration is absolutely crucial to the continued growth of the body. This regeneration process however, often excludes scar tissue.

When you type on your computer, scratch an itch, catch a football, or eat a sandwich, whether or not it hurts, you are causing micro-tears in muscle and connective tissue. Within milliseconds of any body movement, your body is rushing chemicals and cells to an area to create repairs in that area. In our Western society, we tend to think of our bodies as being relatively simple, relatively stagnant, and we don't take any notice of the healing process until we really hurt ourselves.

That is probably why you bought this book in the first place, because you burned your hand with an iron, had a surgery which caused a large trauma in your body, or perhaps you won an award for the best overall free fall and crash on the bunny slope at a mountain resort.

In any case, my point is that the body is not stagnant until we injure it. It is a constantly moving, growing, regenerating city that likes to move. In fact, cities that never sleep - (Las Vegas, New York, Tokyo, Paris, etc.) have nothing on the human body system. If we are engaged in proper activities to take care of our bodies, our cities function in ways that civic planners can only dream about.

In the body, our traffic jams are quickly resolved, our damaged roads are quickly repaired, and our catastrophes are healed overnight. Our bodies are like cities, and we, as conscious beings, are like the giant fuel source. The more we move, the more healthfully we eat, the more good clean oxygen we breathe, the more we encourage our bodies to try new things, and the more we grow our minds, the more healthy our bodies will be. If we can remember this as we go about our daily activities, scar tissue healing, and healing in general, will come much easier to us.

TIME FOR CREATION

As stated above, think about your body like a huge city that constantly regenerates itself. There are millions of little tiny machines all over the body, called cells, which are constantly performing tasks designed to aid the body in growth and development.

These little machines run all around your body. Many of them have very specific tasks and duties to perform. These cells in the body are like the blue and white collar workers in a city. They go to the same locations, do the same tasks, and generally repeat this process over and over until their retiring day.

(Some of them, however, we overwork, and don't take care of through nutrition. These cells sometimes think that they have to keep working, because they're broke, and haven't been able to receive or process the information well enough over their life-span to realize that it's time to let go or give up. This is one of the causes of cancer, but that is a bigger topic that won't be gone into in this book.)

There are other cells which are more like the inventors and the scientists in a city. Just like in an actual city, there are not as many of the scientist/inventor cells, but they create the pathways and the means by which the worker cells do their jobs.

Scar tissue is the result of scientist cells working together with worker cells to heal trauma to the body.

According to Merriam-Webster, (the online version), scar tissue is: the connective tissue forming a scar, and composed chiefly of[1] fibroblasts in recent scars and largely of dense collagenous fibers in old scars.

Brittanica.com defines a scar as:

> A mark left on the skin after a wound heals. Cells called fibroblasts produce collagen fibers, which form bundles that make up the bulk of scar tissue. Scars have a blood supply but no oil glands or elastic tissue, so they can be slightly painful or itchy. Hypertrophic scars grow overly thick and fibrous but remain within the original wound site. Scars can also develop into tumor-like growths called keloids, which extend beyond the wound's limits. Both can inhibit movement when they result from serious burns over large areas, especially around a joint. Scars, especially those from unaided healing of third-degree burns, can become malignant... As part of the healing process, specialized cells called fibroblasts, in adjacent areas of skin, produce a fibrous connective tissue made up of collagen. The bundles formed[2] these whitish, rather inelastic fibers make up the bulk of the scar by tissue.

Both sources mention collagen and fibroblasts, so let's go a little more in-depth about each of them.

Fibroblasts:
Fibroblasts according to Webster are a connective-tissue cell of mesenchymal origin that secretes proteins and especially molecular collagen from which the extracellular fibrillar matrix of connective tissue forms. [1]

 HUH?

Okay - this time in English. Fibroblasts are "scientist" cells which let out proteins (mostly collagen). This collagen builds connections all over the place, particularly across the scar, and that helps connective tissue to grow. When the scar is fully healed, it becomes much more like regular skin, with regular nerve pathways ('worker' cells travel these pathways), regular blood flow (for white and red blood 'worker' cells to reach the area), and natural elasticity and movement.

(Hopefully this definition is a little easier to understand!)

Fibroblasts (according to Encyclopedia Brittanica) are large, flat, elongated (spindle-shaped) cells possessing processes extending out from the ends of the cell body. The cell nucleus is flat and oval. Fibroblasts produce tropocollagen, which is the forerunner of collagen, and ground substance, an amorphous, gel-like matrix that fills the spaces in-between. (2)

Again, reading this can make your brain just totally go to sleep. At least it did mine the first few times I read it. The funniest part of the definition is that, if you'll read closely, you'll read the term 'ground substance.' That's the scientific term for "we pretty much don't know what the heck to call this stuff, and the guy who discovered it has a really long and difficult to pronounce name, so we'll just call it… ummm…. Substance. Yah, that's it! And it kind of looks like it's ground, so, we'll call it ground substance!"

Joking aside, the importance of fibroblasts can't be overstated. They're involved in normal growth, healing, wound repair, and the day-to-day activities of every tissue and organ in the body. The fibroblast does everything. Fibroblasts can de-differentiate back to earlier stages in their development and then re-differentiate into some other cell type.

For you, this would be like waking up one day when you're, oh, let's say, 92, and deciding that by tomorrow, you would like to be 20 again. If you were a fibroblast, you would just do that. (Now, there are people in their fifties who seem like they're in their twenties, in activity and in appearance. Those people have learned how to tap into the changing power of their bodies through health and nutrition. But that is a topic for a different book.)

The fibroblast is seen here *en face*, that is, looking down on it from the top. The sketch shows a little more clearly the nature of the cell.
Fibroblasts are flattened, and like this one, usually have a spiky and irregular outline. They're sometimes referred to as "stellate" in shape, from the Latin word *stella*, meaning "star." You will note that there are some wispy extensions of the cell's cytoplasm. These "arms" are

sitting on collagen fibers (which(5) mostly invisible in this image) and acting to are maintain and repair those fibers.

Fibroblasts are recognizable by three main things.

Number one is their shape. We kind of just covered that, and as you might already be getting bored by the science stuff herein, I will not restate what has been said already

Secondly, fibroblasts are identified by their large complement of RER (RER is Rough Endoplasmic Reticulum. Endoplasmic reticulum is a network of tubules, vesicles and sacs that are interconnected. They may serve specialized functions in the cell including protein synthesis, sequestration of calcium, production of steroids, storage and production of glycogen, and insertion of membrane proteins.)

Finally, Fibroblasts have a large, prominent nucleolus when they're actively making materials.

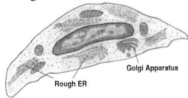

Interference with their activities causes a vast array of clinical problems. The deficiency affects a specific pathway in collagen creation, with consequences ranging from skin sores, anemia, edema, ulcerated gums, loosened teeth, and hemorrhage of mucous membranes. Restoration of) the vitamin allows the fibroblasts to work normally and cures the problem. (5

Collagen

Collagen is the structural protein of bones, tendons, ligaments, and skin. A precursor of collagen called pro(2)ollagen is converted in the c body into collagen .

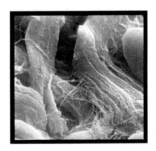

About one quarter of all of the protein in your body is collagen. Collagen is a major structural protein, forming molecular cables that strengthen the tendons, and vast, resilient sheets that support the skin and internal organs. Bones and teeth are made by adding

mineral crystals to collagen. Collagen provides structure to our bodies, protecting and supporting the softer tissues and connecting them with the skeleton. But, in(3) spite of its critical function in the body, collagen is a relatively simple protein.

Hydroxyproline, which is critical for collagen stability, is created by modifying some standard amino acids after the collagen chain is built. The reaction requires vitamin C, which assists with oxygen in the process. Unfortunately, none of us make vitamin C within our bodies, and if we don't get enough Vitamin C in our diet, the results can be disastrous. Vitamin C deficiency slows the production of hydroxyproline and stops the construction of new collagen, ultimately causing scurvy. The symptoms of scurvy-loss of teeth and easy bruising-are caused(3) the lack of collagen to repair the wear-and-tear caused by by everyday activities.

When the body needs to build any new cellular structure, as in the healing process, collagen and/or collagen fragments play a central role. Although the role of collagen as scaffolding has been known for some time, we now know that collagen controls cell shape and differences in cells. It also controls the cells' ability to move through the body, and it aids in the cell's ability create a number of proteins. This is why broken bones regenerate and wounds heal. This is also why blood vessels grow to feed healing areas. The collagen mesh provides the blueprint for what the tissue will look like, the road map for the cells to find where they need to regenerate and grown, and the way for the body to be able to re-grow damaged or broken tissue.

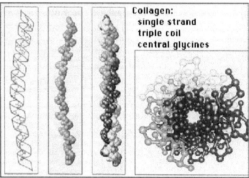

Collagen:
single strand
triple coil
central glycines

Image found on Web identical to Lehninger textbook image, creator unknown.

"OKAY, this is all very interesting. But why do I have scar tissue?"

In short, because scar tissue is necessary for the body to re-grow itself, which it needs to do every day, in order to deal with the wear and tear we put it through.

Hey, Don't Touch Me! Page 12

Here are the really important points to remember about collagen and collagen production:
- Getting a healthy amount of a good source of Vitamin C is important for proper collagen production.
- Getting enough good, clean oxygen into the body is crucial for the chemical change of collagen into other building compounds for the body.
- Collagen acts like scaffolding for our bodies, and it controls the shape and diversity of cells.
- It is why broken bones regenerate and wounds heal.
- It is also why and how blood vessels grow to feed healing areas.

So now that we've learned how scar tissue is created, we should talk about the tissues in the body that the scar tissue affects. These are namely, skin and muscle.

We're going to first talk about muscles.

It's very funny to me how in the English language, we use the word "push" to describe many different types of movement:

- I can push something physically (As in "Monkey Man pushed the car.")
- I can push something emotionally (As in "Monkey Man pushed me into it, even though I didn't want to do it.")
- I can push something to a new plane (As in "Monkey Man's workout took him to a whole new level!")

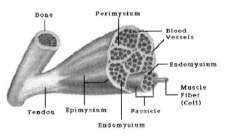

One additional way we use the word push is to describe the action of a muscle. We say "Push your arms together." This is a totally inaccurate statement. Muscles never push, they only pull. In other words, you don't get any force from your body when your muscles relax, you only get force from your body when muscles contract. This is important because when you talk about healing scar tissue within muscle tissue, it's important you understand that your muscles really only have one real movement they can do.

That movement is to contract. The other thing they have the ability to do is relax. So let's talk for a minute about muscle tissue.

The pictures you're looking at have a ton of names and really scientific terms used to describe muscle tissue.

It's not necessary that you know any of these names. In fact, if you never learn any of them, you're probably going to be glad that you didn't cloud your brain with the information that you didn't need to begin with.

What is important is that you gain an understanding of the structure of muscles, and if you decide to call something that I talk about some ridiculous name to help you remember it, like norfgeblatic machilisium, (my made up name), then no problem at all, if that works for you to remember what it is. Like I said, the most important part of all of this is for you to gain an understanding of how muscle tissue and muscle cells work. I'm going to talk about them here with some help from Eastern Kentucky University's Department of Biology [7].

Structure of Skeletal Muscle:

Skeletal muscles are usually attached to bone by tendons composed of connective tissue. This connective tissue also covers the entire muscle & is called epimysium. *(See what I mean about funky names of stuff. Don't get hung up on the terms. Just get an understanding of what the muscle looks like.)*

Skeletal muscles consist of numerous bundles, called fasicles (or fascicles). Fascicles are also surrounded by connective tissue (called the perimysium) and each fascicle is composed of numerous muscle fibers (or muscle cells). Muscle cells, which are wrapped by endomysium, consist of many fibrils (or myofibrils), and these myofibrils are made up of long protein molecules called

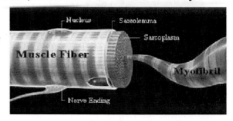

myofilaments.

The cell membrane of a muscle cell is called the sarcolemma, and this membrane, like that of neurons, maintains a membrane potential. So, impulses travel along muscle cell membranes just as they do along nerve cell membranes. However, the 'function' of impulses in muscle cells is to cause the muscle to contract.

Whoa! That was a lot take in. Can you explain that again in a different way?

Sure! Thanks for asking! Here's another way of looking at this.

Imagine you are a city planner. You have been assigned the project of managing all of the city's utilities. So, being the smart person you are, you decide to use big elastic pipes (like the normal metal ones used for getting water to an entire city for plumbing, only you make the pipe stretchy). You're going to put this big pipe next to other big pipes, or other hard objects like dirt and rocks (in the case of the body; bones, organs, etc.), and you want to protect it, so you wrap it in a plastic protective coating (kind of like an insulation).

BIG PIPE
A.K.A. Muscle

Inside of the big elastic pipe are different groups of smaller elastic pipes. You want to protect each group from each other group, so you wrap each group in something protective.

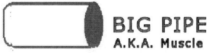

Fassicles
A.K.A. Smaller pipes

Within each group, are individual pipes. Now all of these pipes can move separately from each other, so you're going to want to make sure that they work together, and don't rub against eachother, so you're going to wrap each one in some kind of protective coating, which is also stretchy.

Muscle Fibers
A.K.A. Individual Pipes

Now here's where the body gets different than the pipe example. In city planning, different pipes do different things. Some of them carry hot water, some cold water, some of them carry waste products (Add extra insulation to those! We don't want them to break!), some carry electricity, some carry high speed communications cables.

The human body is a thousand times more sophisticated than even the most sophisticated city. In the human body, the muscle fibers are made up of muscle cells. That means that inside each muscle fiber are muscle cells. Each muscle cell:

- needs fresh blood (with new clean oxygen)
- needs to have waste carried away
- needs to be able to receive and transmit electric impulses

Each of the muscle fibers also has to be able to carry materials and messages in both directions.

So what could prevent the movement of blood, or messages, through the muscle fibers? Anything. If an area is cut, or severely bruised, or misused, or not used, it can develop a situation where blood flow is no longer able to get through, messages are no longer able to be carried, and waste is no longer able to be removed.

In the case of a physical trauma to an area, specific kinds of cells (the earlier mentioned fibroblasts) go through the process of creating a map, for other cells to come in and create new tissue. Sometimes this tissue heals completely and becomes new skin. Other times, the tissue isn't able to create all the necessary physical pathways due to distance, or lack of movement in an area. As a result, the tissue hardens and turns into what we know as scar tissue.

So, in review:

Fibroblasts: Cells with incredible skills. They lay the foundation, or scaffolding, if you will, for tissue growth.

Collagen: Collagen is the structural protein of bones, tendons, ligaments, and skin.

Fassicles: Groups of muscle fibers

Muscle Fibers: muscle cells in long strands within a fassicle, within the muscle itself.

"OKAY! OKAY! I get it!"
"Stop with the definitions already! I understand all of that. I didn't get your book so that I could take a test! I agree that by reading further, I already know that
- nutrition is a key in healing scar tissue.
- the body must go through a process of healing which can take some time, in order to heal the scar tissue fully.
- muscles don't push, they pull. This means that I will need to re-teach my body how to unite groups of muscle fibers so that they work together, particularly in areas where there has been a trauma which caused scar tissue, but also throughout my body in general.

I understand all of that. What I really want to know about **my** scar tissue is:"
WHY IS IT SO LUMPY?

The natural regeneration powers of higher mammals is poor. We're not like lizards or other amphibians. We can't regenerate limbs. So don't go hacking your hand off thinking it will grow back. It won't. Sorry!

However, we can regenerate our blood, our liver (as long as a quarter of it remains intact), our outer most skin layer, and fingertips from the base of the nail upwards. The mechanism of regeneration is well known and is triggered by a flow of DC current from the severed nerve endings to the neuroepidermal junctions (The place where the brain monitors what's going on) in the skin.

So let's get into your skin now (Hey, it's better than getting under your skin. Okay, cheesy joke. My apologies).

Skin is one of the most amazing organs of the human body. It is hard for us to think about it as an organ, however. We tend to think of organs as boxy things. Your heart, liver, kidneys - those are obviously organs. But skin is an organ too.

Skin is made up of very specific cells and tissues, and their collective purpose is to act as the boundary between "you" and "the world". One of the neat things about skin that makes it different from a lot of other organs is the fact that it does have to deal with the real world. Therefore it is loaded with sensors, and it also has a very tough layered design, so that it can handle the realities of the environment like cuts and sunlight.

Here's a diagram to help you see what is going on. If you take a look at a cross-section of typical skin (like the skin on your arm or leg) you find that it is made up of two main layers: the epidermis on the outside and the dermis on the inside. The epidermis is the barrier, while the dermis is the layer containing all the "equipment" - things like nerve endings, sweat glands, hair follicles and so on.

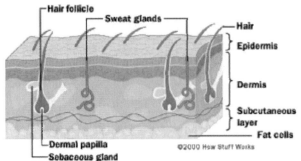

In the subcutaneous layer (you may have heard of subcutaneous fat - this is where it hides) you can see the blood vessels (shown as two thin red and blue lines). These vessels branch infinitely (not shown) into the dermis to supply the sweat glands, hair follicles, sebaceous glands and erector muscles with blood. They also fan out into the dermis's capillary bed. It turns out that the dermis is loaded with capillaries. Capillaries satisfy the nutritional needs of the cells in the dermis, and they also help the skin perform an important cooling function in humans. The epidermis has no direct blood supply, but instead is supported and fed by the dermis.

The dermis is where the action is for body functions. As shown in the diagram, the dermis contains sweat glands, hair follicles (each with its own tiny little muscle so that your "hair can stand on end"!), nerve endings, etc. There are several different types of nerve endings:

- Heat sensitive
- Cold sensitive
- Pressure sensitive • Itch sensitive • Pain sensitive

All these different nerve endings let you sense the world. They also help you protect yourself from burns, punctures, etc. by warning you when something is damaging your skin.

The epidermis is your interface to the world, and it is actually quite interesting. It has two main layers, the inner of which is living and the outer of which is dead. The dead skin cells of the outer layer are what we can actually see, and they are constantly flaking off and being replaced by new cells being pushed outward. This happens about every 30 days.

The living, inner layer is called the malpighian layer. The malpighian layer creates the dead cells that we can see. It is in direct contact with the dermis, which feeds and supports it.

Next up is something called the stratum corneum. (*more complex scientific names*!) This is the outer layer of dead cells - the cells that we see as our skin. The cells in this layer are filled with a protein called keratin. Keratin is a very interesting protein because it is very solid and strong. Horns, hair, hoofs, fingernails and feathers all gain their strength from keratin. The same stuff that your fingernails are made of actually forms your visible skin. That is what makes your skin so tough. In parts of the body that get a lot of wear, like the palms and the feet, the stratum corneum is thicker. (12)

So let's go back to the dermis layer with its hair follicles and nerve cells.

Pathcurve.com states that "nerves are sheathed in a perineural sleeve of schwann cells which supply the nerves stimulus, essential to regeneration."

?????

Yah, Me too. I was very confused the first time I read it.

Here's a translation of what pathcurve.com told us just a second ago: Remember the pipe example, the one where you're the city planner? Well, nerves work the exact same way, except that the pipe is a collection of what are known as schwann cells.

Pathcurve.com goes on to say that:

"When a nerve is severed, provided that the schwann cells are able to reconnect (they can grow over small distances) then

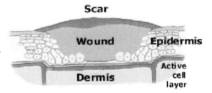

regeneration and complete healing takes place. But when the wound or cut or damage is quite bad and no electrical conductivity can be re-established between the cut nerve and the neuroepidermal cell into which it "plugs", then regeneration cannot take place and the rapid build up of collagen is necessary to plug the hole.

"Because collagen is produced in abundance by fibroblasts, it invariably forms a domed layer over the wound and this domed layer is the scar which is often disfiguring and large.

"There are few, if any, neuroepidermal junctions in scar tissue so it has very little touch sensation. Because of this, the mind, which perceives the body as a hologram of nerve endings, doesn't send much blood to the area of scar tissue, so it doesn't stay very supple and doesn't grow. This means that it doesn't regenerate like the rest of the skin, otherwise it would fall off and renew like the rest of the skin." [6]

OUCH! THAT HURTS!

Another issue of scar tissue is that the surrounding skin tends to be much more sensitive than normal healthy skin.

Imagine this…If you were a nerve, you would be going along, minding your own business, and suddenly, you would bump up against all the other cells and materials who had to stop because of the trauma up ahead.

Another way to state this is this. Imagine you are driving down a highway, through the middle of nowhere, in your SUV. Up ahead, the bridge has washed out. You can't go back because there's too much traffic behind you and no way to turn around. Plus, you have to get to your destination. So, you go four-wheeling on a jeep trail to the nearest town. Well, in that town, there is a bridge across the river, and it only takes you 20 minutes longer to get to your destination. So, even though you know a shorter route, you decide to always take the road through the town, because the people are friendlier there, and the road there has never washed out, and you just feel more comfortable that way.

In the body, sometimes the "bridge" never is repaired. So often, the cut or damaged nerves re-route to the nearest area of normal skin and plug into healthy skin cells there.

This can make the skin around any scar more sensitive and often quite painful for longer periods of time. This is also what leads to the zinging electric feeling that often accompanies scars when you touch them.

---Key point---

This zinging feeling is an important feeling to pay attention to, and mentally, it's important to let those nerves try to create a new bridge into, and across, the forming scar.

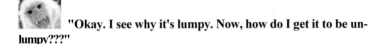 **"Okay. I see why it's lumpy. Now, how do I get it to be un-lumpy???"**

That is what the rest of this book covers!

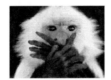

Physiology and Psychology

As far as the actual actions you will take after reading this book, there are two kinds of activities. There are the physical activities of healing the scar tissue (things like specific movements and eating well), and there are mental activities that you will be asked to engage in.

Healing, depending on whom you talk to, is a complex process. Some people believe that prayer alone will heal, while others believe that only pills and western medicine will heal. Some have great success with acupuncture, others with chiropractic, and others with nutrition. I believe that healing is a combination of all of these things.

Scar tissue healing takes time, and because of that, it takes patience. Patience is the kind of mental activity that will be required of you for healing.

Another is belief. You wouldn't be reading this book if you didn't believe you could heal your scar tissue. You are to be congratulated for taking your healing into your own hands. It will be important for you to maintain a solid level of belief as you work to heal your scar tissue. Belief is the most important factor in any endeavor, whether it be:
- Religion ("If a person has faith the size of a mustard seed, he or she can move mountains." Jesus)
- History ("They can conquer who believe they can." Virgil)
- Science ("In the province of the mind, what one believes to be true either is true or becomes true." John Lilly)
- Healing ("The body needs to adapt itself to the mind. This is why the consideration of belief systems is so important to healing." (Schwartz))

It's not just in my head!

You are absolutely correct. Healing only begins with thoughts in the mind. After that, you will need to take action to get the results you want. What I am trying to encourage you to think about is what is known as BE - DO - HAVE.

If you want to HAVE a more flexible scar, or want to HAVE scar-free skin, then you will need to DO certain activities. These will vary from scar to scar and from person to person. But before doing these activities, you have to decide to BE the kind of person who will be patient and persistent enough to DO what you need to.

Many people think that scar tissue will simply go away after time, and in many cases it does. However, scar tissue is the healing that happens after an injury. It needs to be worked with, using massage, belief, and whatever other methods achieve positive results without further damage, in order to re-heal as effectively as possible.

What I offer here is advice on how to massage scar tissue, with the hope that you will be able to use it and effectively break up your scar tissue. I hope this works for you, and hope as well that you will let me know your results via email at massage@strive4impact.com. I hope you'll incorporate whatever else works for you, as that will help speed up your healing.

Part II. "Hey, I Need to Know!"

Can this really work?
How can I massage or work with my scar tissue

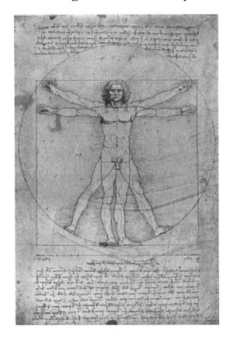

Can this really work?

Like anything, healing works when you work at it. However, unlike anything else, healing will work for you (at least for a time), when you're not working at it. The human body is such an amazing machine, with the ability to produce everything it needs, so long as we give it the materials and the right environment for healing.

In this section, you will learn specific techniques for working with specific muscles and parts of the body.

For some parts of the body, there are specific movements and exercises you will want to do. However, there are many general hand positions and techniques which will apply for many situations and many different parts of the body. Those definitions and techniques are defined and demonstrated here.

When scar tissue develops, the brain/nerve connections, which have to happen to detect touch, never develop or develop very weak. This is because scar tissue develops primarily to heal and protect, and only secondarily to feel sensation. In other words, the tissue naturally develops a weak ability to notice sensation while it is being created. Because most people don't use or touch a part of the body which had a kind of trauma to it, (like that which comes from surgery or a car accident,) the tissue doesn't receive any stimulation.

This means that in many cases (after surgery or other trauma), the secondary function of scar tissue, sensation, never or barely develops. Over time, this lack of sensation causes an area to be touched less (after all, why would a person touch an area that had no feeling?). It receives less touch, and because of this, it receives less stimulation, which means that the nerve endings and connections develop less, which means that the area has less feeling, so it is touched less; and the process goes on until there is a thick mass of non-sensory tissue, most of it probably scar tissue.

In the deeper layers of skin tissue, it is important to know that just as scar tissue develops on the outside layers of the skin, it develops in the muscle. Muscle can be divided into two groups with regard to scar tissue; areas which can be worked through direct massage, and those which are much more difficult to work with using massage. Most massage therapists have developed an ability to work at a deep level within the muscle that most non massage therapists have not. For the areas which are difficult to get to when doing massage yourself, I would recommend getting into a regular stretching program and getting regular massage. Most recreation/fitness centers now offer Yoga classes. If yours doesn't offer Yoga or another kind of stretching program, ask them why they don't, and consider joining one that does.

Also, consider getting regular scar tissue massage for a while. If you don't know a good massage therapist, ask a friend who gets regular massage, or even look up a CMT in the phone book. You can find criteria for selecting a massage therapist by clicking here. You may have to take some time researching, but it will be worth it when you find a therapist with whom you feel comfortable, and schedule an appointment. Massage can range from $20 to upwards of $300/hour. The cost doesn't necessarily determine the quality of the massage, so don't think you have to pay an arm and a leg to get a great massage. Let the therapist know your wants with regard to getting your scar tissue broken up, and they should be able to help you. If your goal is getting your scar tissue broken up, ask for a massage therapist who specializes in Neuro Muscular Rehabilitation (NMR), or a comparable technique.

That's enough about selecting a massage therapist. You've decided to take your healing into your own hands, and this section will help you do just that.

Point/Prick method
GOAL: Re-establish sensation (nerve pathways) into the scar tissue.

To deal with the tissue that isn't sensing touch very well, use the point/prick method. This can most often be done when you find yourself in a setting where you only need to listen to what's going on. Take a sharpened pencil, paper clip, nail file, or even a needle (something with a small point), and see what kind of feeling you have in a specific spot on the scar. Really pay attention to what kinds of sensations you have in the spot that you're touching. Make sure you don't pierce the skin, as that would only cause further injury to a healing area. However, make sure to test and see how much sensation you have.

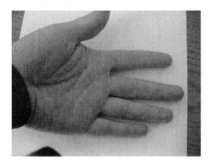

A personal note: This is my huge hand - probably one of the reasons I am a massage therapist is because of my huge hands. Or, maybe I have huge hands because I am a massage therapist. (Look Mom! I'm famous! My hand is in a book!)

Notice the scars on my middle and fourth fingers. These scars on my fingers came from a surgery I had in September of 1994. I have used the point/prick technique on this scar since then. I wish I had a before and after picture to show you how much the scar tissue has gone away, but you will just have to take my word for it. Over time, the sensations have become stronger and more definite in the scar tissue itself, and as the sensation has come back, the scar tissue has been reduced (not gone away), and become much less painful. It probably also helps that I am a massage therapist, and while working on a client, I use the sensations coming from my hands to understand when a muscle is tight, or when it has knots, etc. I pay a lot of attention to the sensations coming from my fingers. You can do the same with scars anywhere on your body. That is the idea of the point/prick method.

Physical Activity:

Touch the scar with an object with a small point in several specific spots on and around the scar. Can you feel the sensation? If not, start by going around the edge of the scar. Can you feel that sensation? Notice what it feels like. Does it make a difference if you press hard or light? What about if you move it around a little? What about if you lightly scrape across the scar (Not piercing the skin, just lightly going across it)?

Mental Activity:

Set an intention that you want to feel sensation in that specific point you are touching. By doing this, and focusing your attention on it, you are forcing your brain and your body to focus in on the sensory information you should be receiving from those nerves.

Just like working to develop more flexibility by stretching the same muscles over an extended amount of time, you are working to develop those nerves, and regenerate them if necessary, on a daily basis, by using different kinds of touch. Over time, you will redevelop more feeling in the area than you previously had.

Let your brain reconnect with this part of your body. If you can begin to feel sensation within small points in the scar, or around the scar, then there is a nerve pathway somewhere in the area. You can help this nerve pathway to branch through the scar (over time), and can get more sensation back into the area. This will lead to the brain reconnecting with this tissue, which will ultimately re-establish blood flow to the area.

Cross-Fibering Method
GOALS:

- Release toxins stored in the muscle tissue.
- Break down small adhesions in the muscle which don't belong there.
- Encourage the formation of strong, pliable scar tissue at the site of healing injuries.
- Reduce the roughness that forms between tendons and their sheaths that can result in painful tendonitis.
- Prevent or soften adhesions in the muscle tissue/tendon.
- The idea with cross-fibering is to work across the direction that the muscle tissue naturally lays. You can do this with any muscle.

Start by using a cream, lotion, or oil (I personally recommend Lotus Touch cream, available from www.lotustouch.com) and use it on the area you want to work. Skinstore.com also sells a few creams and gels, which have been reported to help considerably to diminish the tightness and the overall thickness of scar tissue. Remember that you are using the massage cream to allow your hands or a tool to more easily move across the skin, so if the skin soaks all of it up, you may need to reapply. You will then want to work across the muscle fibers.

For example, let's look at the muscles around the knee: as you are standing, most of the muscle fibers go up and down, so you will want to work across the leg. You can use massage tools and/or implements to get into the muscle deeply and work across the muscle, or you can use your hands. One good hand position is shown in the picture. Using this hand position, use the second knuckle (closest knuckle to the hand) on the middle and ring fingers, to get into the muscle fibers of the quads/calves, while the second and pinky fingers glide across the leg. Move up and down the muscle, making sure to focus on areas where it feels like there is more binding of the tissues. You can finish by doing a gentle massage on the area to calm it down. This is one possibility for cross-fibering.

Whatever hand position or tool you use with cross-fibering, remember that your goal is to break up the scar tissue by going across the muscle, and remember that this isn't going to happen overnight. By using cross-fibering, you are actually causing minor traumas to an area which promote the healing in that area. You don't want to re-injure the area to the point where more scar tissue develops because of your working on it. A generally good way to know how much pressure is enough is that it should be on the level between uncomfortable and painful. So it should be uncomfortable, but not overly painful. As far as the time it takes for healing, a good general guideline is that you should give the scar tissue as long to break up (if you're working on it daily) as it did for it to be created. In other words, if you had surgery two years ago, and you just started working with the scar tissue yesterday, large improvements could take up to two years from yesterday. Healing doesn't have to take this long, but this should give you an idea of how patient you should be.

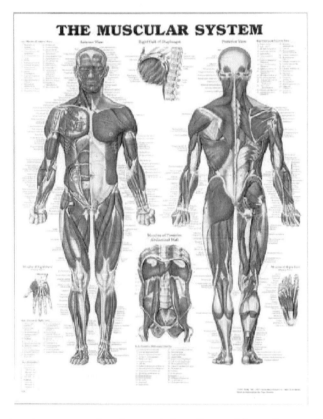

This chart is not comprehensive, nor is it really very big on the page. The point in showing you this chart is to give you an idea of how cross-fibering works.

On the front side (anterior), if you want to work the Pectoralis Major (that is the breast muscle tissue), then to cross-fiber this muscle, you would work from the shoulder toward the sternum. On the back side (posterior), If you wanted to work the Gluteus Maximus (better known as the butt), you would work from the hip towards the upper portion of the inside of the leg.

The Pinch method

(Notice how I love really technical terms? I figure that if I use a term you can understand, rather than making up some overly complicated technical term, then we will all be better off.)

Goals:

- Assess the amount of scar tissue in an area
- Establish sensation in an area
- Loosens the connective tissue around the outside of the scar
- This possibly may be painful in areas of restriction

Physical activity of the Pinch Method

Basically, the pinch method is exactly what it sounds like. Take the area of skin you want to work on, and pinch it between your forefinger and thumb, or between two fingers, or between your hands.

Then you will want to do what is called skin rolling.

Skin rolling is also what it sounds like. While the skin is pinched, roll it back and forth. The purpose of this is to increase blood flow in the area, while encouraging the tissue to relax, loosen up, and allow the nerve cells to push back through the scar.

Mental Activity of the Pinch Method

While you are pinching and rolling, get your brain involved.

Notice how the scar tissue feels. Is it more solid than the rest of your skin? Is it more loose than the rest of your skin? Does it have more or less feeling than the rest of your skin? Get very specific and detailed about your observations. You could even keep a journal of these observations every day, to track your progress and to show how you are improving over time.

Effleurage/Petrissage method
Goals:

- Flushing toxins through the body
- Increasing blood flow
- Opening glands and pores which may be blocked
- Stimulate sensory nerve endings to bring a reflex response in the skin's circulatory network.
- Create a feeling of relaxation, which can be healing in and of itself.

Effleurage is a rhythmic stroking motion. For example, effleurage of the abdomen is used in the Lamaze method of childbirth, in order to sooth and calm the mother (and potentially, the father too!). Petrissage is a deeper kind of skin massage where the skin is gently lifted and squeezed.

These techniques are better known as Swedish massage, which is, contrary to popular belief, a lighter kind of massage aimed at loosening tension in the skin and outer layers of muscle.

The pressure used varies according to the underlying muscle, skin, and tone, but the pressure is not designed to break up tissue as much as encourage blood flow and sensation through stroking and squeezing.

The hand contours to the skin with the idea being that the maximum part of the surface of the palm should be in contact with the body. At the same time, even pressure, rhythm, and rate of movement are used to achieve a calming effect.

Using these techniques:

- point/prick
- cross-fibering
- Pinch Method/skin rolling
- Effleurage/Petrissage

You should find that over time, you can work through the scar tissue and begin to get feeling back in the area. So now we get into the nitty-gritty!

 "Finally!"

What we are going to cover here is specific bodywork for the following areas.
- knees
- elbows
- face
- abdominal
- uterine • breast
- back
- shoulder
- extremities
- other

Remember as we go through this, that when the methods above are talked about, they are talked about with the understanding that you will be doing BOTH, the physical AND mental activity of the method. There is a tendency for people to just do the physical activity, but getting the brain involved is crucial to scar tissue healing.

There are two general kinds of massage you can do for any part of the body. These types are really complex, so are you ready? The two types of massage are:
The kind of massage you give to yourself
The kind of massage someone else gives you.

I will try to cover both, but might not be able to offer suggestions for ways you can work on yourself for all parts of the body. For instance, it is kind of difficult to give yourself a back massage, and even more difficult to give yourself a gluteal massage (that's the butt, in case you were wondering). But I will make some suggestions for things you can try on your own for these areas that are hard to reach.

Just a general rule, which would seem to go without saying, but I will say it anyway - a good hand washing is always a good idea before giving massage. We carry a significant amount of bacteria on our hands. And if you are to be the receiver of massage, make sure that your body is clean, and that you've taken the time to have good hygiene. Someone is being nice enough to work on your body, so show your appreciation by being clean.

Most importantly, be patient, get your mind involved with your body, and let's show you how to heal scar tissue anywhere in your body!

The Knees

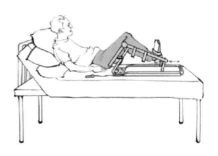

It's only fitting that we should begin with the knees. These are some of the most troublesome spots for people. I know from my own experience with ACL surgery, that the recovery process can be long, and can be frustrating. But it is also very rewarding to have a great knee today, and one that moves freely and without pain!

See this? This is called a CPM unit (CPM = Continuous Passive Movement). I highly recommend that if you haven't yet had your ACL surgery, you look into having one of these immediately after recovery. If your surgeon or physical therapist says that they don't like CPM units because they like to keep the knee immobilized after ACL surgery, I would recommend you find a new surgeon. This may come across as harsh or unrealistic, but in the case of a ligament reattachment, where the tendons are holding the joint together, movement is much better than non-movement. There are rare exceptions where you would want the knee to be immobilized after knee surgery, but really, keeping the knee immobilized isn't a good idea. The recovery takes longer, and the surgery is generally less effective.

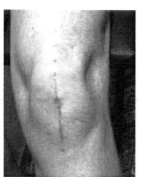

I'm not talking about all knee surgeries, just ACL surgeries.

When it comes to the knees, scar tissue can be a real challenge, because if you want to walk, thick scar tissue can be a real impediment to doing so. Plus, knees are in a visible place, and as some of the pictures on the knees pages show, scars on knees can be large, and rather unfriendly looking.

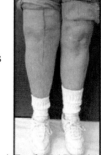

Hey, Don't Touch Me! Page 36

"In athletes, soft tissue pain in the retinaculum (tendon tissue) of the anterior (front of the knee) is fairly common. This may come from strain of the tendon - which connects the kneecap to the lower leg bone (patellar tendon), upper leg bone (quadriceps tendon), or the retinaculum (which supports the kneecap on both the left and right sides.)

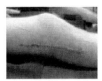

Some pain in the knee is caused by the kneecap being abnormally aligned. If the patella is not correctly aligned, it may come under excessive stress, particularly with vigorous activities. This can also cause excessive wear on the cartilage of the kneecap, which can result in chondromalacia (a condition in which the cartilage softens and may cause a painful sensation in ai the underlying bone or irritation of the synovium [joint lining].) If you suspect this is the case for you, try first loosening the muscles and tendons using the techniques outlined here. If that isn't working and you're still having pain, talk with your doctor to see what can be done.

What you can do for yourself:
Stretching, pinch method, point/prick method, effleurage, petrissage

One simple stretch is to lie on your stomach, grab the ankle of the affected leg with one hand, and gently stretch the front of the knee by pulling the ankle to a level that is uncomfortable.

If your scar tissue is right over the knee cap, you'll probably have to lift it up off of the knee and squeeze it between your thumbs and forefingers to get to it (pinch method). However, if it is in a more substantial set of muscle (lower quads), you will be able to work your fingers across the muscle and use a cross-fiber technique on the muscle (or have someone do this for you).

From a sitting position, place your hands on either side of your leg, with your fingertips touching the point where the upper part of your leg meets the lower part of your leg. Begin by making small circles with your fingers along the sides of your knee, and move up into the thigh. Do some small circles and large circles with your fingers. Do the same small and large circles with your thumbs, going up and down the top of the thigh and noticing what sensations are going through your leg. Try more pressure. Try less pressure. If you push one place, can you feel it pulling somewhere else?

Put your awareness into the muscle you are working on. By doing this type of activity and getting your mind involved, you are encouraging blood to flow more freely through the muscles, carrying away toxins, and bringing in new oxygen and nutrients to power the muscles and nerves.

What someone else can do for you:
Changes may not be immediate, as you are trying to alter mechanical patterns in your body that have been established for some time. However, you should start to feel some improvement within about three to four times of someone working with you.

There can be a lot of extra tension in the muscles surrounding the knee (the quadriceps, hamstrings, gastrocnemius, soleus, and Anterior tibialis, which are known to most of us as thigh, back of thigh, calf, and shin). Getting the body to let go of this tension is an important factor in any kind of knee injury, so massage methods aimed at reducing the tightness in these muscles are helpful. This includes compressive effleurage and deep tissue work. You can also work the muscle in the same direction as the muscle tissue runs. The picture to the right shows a quadriceps 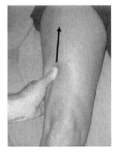 muscle being worked by a therapist's thumb, going in the same direction as the muscle. Depending on the depth at which you work, working in the same direction as the muscle tissue naturally lays can also break up adhesions in the muscle tissue, including scarring.

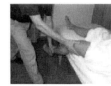 Try using cross-fibering techniques in the muscles and around the tendons. Try doing the cross-fibering in several directions across the muscle. Do this for yourself, let someone else do it for you, or you can use a household tool if you can't get the kind of pressure you want.

Now that might sound funny, "Use a household tool." But really, my family and friends will tell you, I've been caught subconsciously working my forearms out on the edge of a counter, or using a rolling pin/pizza dough roller to roll out stress out of someone's shoulders. Just make sure that your tool, whatever it is, is rounded (not sharp!) and has a good fit with whatever part of the body you're working. (Hint: a rolling pin works very well for working on the quads by yourself.)

Special attention should be paid to any area that has been giving you more pain, especially if that pain is consistent with the pain you have been experiencing related to doing physical activities… walking, running, skiing, hiking, biking, etc.

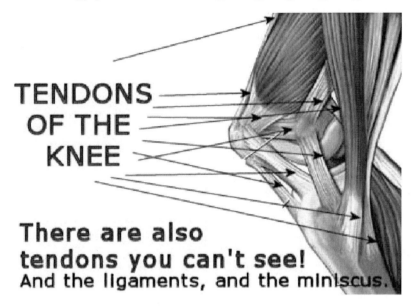

TENDONS OF THE KNEE

There are also tendons you can't see! And the ligaments, and the miniscus.

As you can see, the knee is a very complex thing, as are most joints in the body. Treat it like the complex machine that it is. Pay attention to all the various parts of the knee. It will aid in your healing.

Stretching the muscle groups around the knee is also a very important activity during the rehabilitation process. Now, you're probably heard of a knee stretch somewhere along the way, and if not, do a Google Search for knee stretches. See what you come up with.

What I wanted to do instead is offer you some stretches you may not have thought about or even heard of. Some stretches that you can do with the knees involve the use of a sheet. These can be done by yourself or with the help of a friend or workout partner.

Try these! They're fun and they will help you to heal your knees.

Knee Stretch #1

One stretch you can do is to lay flat on the ground. Place a sheet or pillow case under your knees. Take each end of the sheet, one end in each hand, and slowly pull the sheet toward you, making sure it stays behind your knees. Take a deep breath, and when you breathe out, pull your knees toward your chest. Hold this position for a few breaths and then lower the knees a few inches, releasing the stretch. Now you are in perfect position to do knee stretch two.

Knee Stretch #2

Another stretch you can do will move, open, and stretch the spine. When you are done with Knee Stretch One, allow the knees to gently fall to one side by shifting your hold on the sheet. Don't let the legs fall all the way to the ground; have some control of them as they head to one side. Once you have let the legs go one direction, lean back and pull the knees back up to center and then allow them to drop to the other side.

Knee Stretch #3

This is a great move to receive, when you do it with a partner. Make sure you are on some kind of a slick surface… a massage table works well, but in the absence of that, try a counter or table top. (Just make sure it will hold your weight before getting on it. No need to create more scar tissue!)

Begin the move starting with Knee Stretch #2, with the knees off to the left or the right. Before the person you're working with initiates the move, have them ask you if you are ready to be spun around. If you are ready, take a big breath, and, when you exhale, have your partner quickly walk around your body, pulling from the knees and keeping up the momentum so that you spin in a circle on your back.

See, healing can be fun too! Just like the tire swing when you were a kid! Personally, I never much cared for the tire swing because it always made me a bit queasy. But using this exercise, and doing small half-turns, I get to have fun while stretching. You will too! Give it a shot!

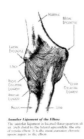

Elbows

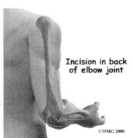

Incision in back of elbow joint

Though never a personal recipient of an elbow injury, I have known and worked with people who have elbow conditions which have not been a lot of fun for them.

Scarring around the elbows can come from a lot of sources, ranging from falls in early childhood to corrective surgeries for adults. In doing the research for this book, I learned that eighty percent of chronic elbow pain actually happens because of a sprain of the annular ligament, which attaches the radius bone to the ulnar bone. Both of those bones are in your forearm, as is the annular ligament. (Just so that you know, ligaments connect bones to bones, while tendons connect muscles to bones.)

"Because of the tremendous demands placed on the fingers and hands to perform repetitive tasks, the annular ligament is stressed every day [...] and [can become] a source of chronic pain. Chronic elbow pain can also be caused by an ulnar collateral ligament sprain. This ligament supports the inside of the elbow and is responsible for holding the ulnar bone to the distal end of the humerus." (8)

 "Ulnar to humer... WHAT?"

Ever whacked your funny bone? It's not very humorous, huh? But it might be the humerus.

 "Very funny..."

Thank-you!

The bone in the upper part of your arm is called the humerus. The distal end is the end of the bone at your elbow, and it connects to the ulna (one of the bones of your forearm). It does this through a ligament called the ulna collateral

Hey, Don't Touch Me! Page 41

ligament. This ligament is one of the things that give you that "Zing" whenever you hit your "funny bone."

Like the knee, the elbow has a lot of movement tied up in it. All of the finger tendons ultimately attach at the elbow, and much of the strength of your hands is determined by the strength of the muscles around your elbow.

So how can you work on scar tissue around the elbow?

What you can do for yourself:
For the skin and the scar tissue itself, use stretching, the pinch method, the point/prick method, effleurage, and petrissage.

Use this google search for elbow stretches. You should come up with some good elbow stretching exercises. In addition, here are some massage techniques other people can do on you (if you're fortunate enough to find someone who will help you with your healing), with pictures and some help from http://www.massagemag.com, which should help you in the process.

What someone else can do for you:

Have them start with a solid pressure effleurage and light cross-fibering. It will help to get rid of some of the general tightness all over in the muscle, and it will also help you to be able to move your arm/elbow more freely.
After this, try having someone use more pressure along the top of the arm, using their thumbs, or the palm of their hand.
Remember, the muscles of the forearm go primarily the same direction as the bones, so try having someone work with the muscles in the direction they run, and then try having them work across the muscle, using some cross-fibering techniques.

As the skin, tendons, and muscles in the arm loosen up over time, you may find that more pressure will work better for you. You should also try moving your hand up and down as someone works on it, because that movement will actually cause the muscles to work, while they are being worked on. This gets your brain involved in the process of reconnecting the nervous system with the muscular system. It will also help your muscles to work in groups that complement each other, rather than as individual muscle fibers.

You also will want the person working on you to focus on the collagen breakdown problems which can happen in the tendons (in addition to the help they're providing by reducing tension in the muscles around the elbow). One thing you can have someone do is locate the "elbow spot." Again, like I've told you before, I'm really technical, and I like using really complicated terms, which is why I call it the "elbow spot" here.

How to locate the "elbow spot": If you bend your arm, with your palm facing down, the "elbow spot" is on the top of the arm, near where the arm bends. It is a spot where a lot of the tendons come together, and if someone applies a good amount of pressure there, you will probably jump right out of the chair you're sitting in. Where the thumb is placed in this picture is pretty darn close to, if not actually on, the spot. This spot can become bound up from repetitive motion or other kinds of forearm 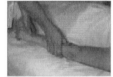 strain, and your tendons can stop the effective production of collagen in this area, due to the binding going on there. In order to break this up, try using the thumb or fingers, and vibrate them back and forth across the muscle tendons in this area of the body.

The amount of pressure should be determined by you, but this is the kind of movement that should use more pressure. Generally speaking, you should be receiving enough pressure that it feels uncomfortable, and even on the verge of painful, but not actually painful. One thing that can be tried is to have the tendons being stretched and relaxed while you are being worked on. This can either be accomplished by you moving your hand up and down at the wrist (using the pulling action of the extensor and flexor muscles in the forearm), or the person working with you can move your hand around for you, perhaps laying your hand across a rolled up towel or something similar. Generally speaking, it will be best if you move your hand to get the stretch, because your brain gets involved that way.

There are other things people can do for you as well. Try combinations of the different techniques offered here to see what works and feels best for you.

Now for more sheet stretches! Have a partner do this one with you as well.

Have the person place the sheet beneath the entire length of one arm. Only the hand should stick out. Have them hold on to each end of the sheet, stand up, and lift until the sheet presses around your arm. Then they will gently twist the sheet ends together, and this will cause the arm to be held inside the sheet completely. The person will stand near your head. Then they gently swing the arm back and forth, out to the side, then up and down. The arm may flop and bend at the elbow. Have the person pull the sheet toward them, and allow the arm to roll back and forth. Then, they will gently lower your arm to the side of your body, and remove the sheet. They can then do the same routine on the other side if they're willing, and if you would like them to.

When the other arm is done, you can move both arms above your head, or they can move your arms for you, and then wrap the sheet loose around your wrists. Then they slowly pull up on your arms using the sheet, which will stretch the shoulder muscles, the skin of the arms, and the elbow joints.

Face

   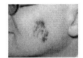

Scar tissue in the Face can often be the thickest of all, not just on a physical level, but on an emotional issue as well.

Images of scarred faces haunt history. There's a great website someone has put together that talks about how Hollywood uses skin disease and scarring to represent evil.

From the web site "Most movies that feature skin disease use it to represent evil. Skin conditions may act as a cinematic shorthand to identify characters that are dangerous or immoral." [14]

Think about people in the history of movies who have had scars on their face to represent how evil they are - there are literally hundreds of examples. Perhaps one of the most prominent is the character of "Johnny" from *Arsenic and Old Lace*, who is the victim of a facial reconstruction gone wrong. This character was played by Boris Karloff and, he was portrayed as extremely evil in the film. (As an aside, *Arsenic and Old Lace* is a great 1930's black and white film and a lot of fun to watch!)

I say all of this, and bring up these points, because if you have facial scarring, you must realize that it is a part of your body. Accept it as something that is a part of your physical make up today. It's the most important thing you can do. Rejecting it as ugly, or evil, or any other such nonsense, will not only cause the area to become more isolated, but such negative mental projection towards this part of your body can actually increase the thickness and severity of the scarring.

- So accept that you have scar tissue in a visible part of your body, and that you would like to get rid of it.
- Also, remember that all positions in life are temporary. You can change the severity of the scar tissue that is visible on your face, and you will if you work with it.

You can change the condition of any physical reality of your body, and if you decide to, you can reduce and even remove any effects of the scar tissue being in such a visible place.

One thing you can start with is a simple facial massage. If you have facial scarring in an area, and it bothers you while doing this activity, work across and through it. Take a minute to notice what there is to notice about the texture of the muscle/skin of the scar tissue, as well as the temperature of the muscle skin in the scar tissue, as it relates to the rest of the surrounding skin.

Now, we will talk about doing a basic facial massage. This entire massage can take a minimum of five minutes, but I've personally seen a facial massage last an hour. The important part is for you to take the time you need, and to let the muscles of your face relax.

- Remember that much of your facial tension can start in the neck and shoulders, so you can start by making firm circular movements, working up both sides of the neck, and then out across the shoulders.
- Using the pads of your fingertips, use a small amount of lotion, or oil, and put it on your forehead, temples, nose, cheeks, chin and ears.
- Make small circles, from the center of each area, and slowly move outward.
- With both hands, if available, you can place the tips of your index, middle and ring fingers closely together on your forehead and rub outward towards the temples, making circular motions and applying gentle pressure.
- Think about the tension we hold around our eyes… Every time you frown, smile, cry, laugh, or express any of the variety of human emotions, there is some expression which happens through the eyes. To release tension around the eyes, firmly squeeze the eyebrows with your thumb and forefinger.
  There are some spa therapists who say that you should always work from the bridge of the nose towards the temples (to prevent wrinkles). I don't know that there is any scientific proof of this, but I put it in here in case that is a concern for you.
- Once again, place the tips of your index, middle and ring fingers close together, except this time place them across the middle of your face, moving in circular motions from the bridge of your nose, across your cheeks, and toward your ears. You can stimulate the skin in the cheeks by using the back of your hands and loosely rolling your fingers up the cheek. This can also be used on the neck and under the chin.

- Put your middle and index fingers together, and place them between your nose and upper lip, moving in circular motions around your mouth. Move down to the hinge of jaw (below and slightly in front of the ears), and massage the jaw area. You will want to massage the Temporo-Mandibular Joint (TMJ), which is the joint where your lower jaw bone is connected to the temporal bone of your skull. It is covered with a thin layer of cartilage and separated by a small disk. This joint is almost constantly in use as you eat, speak and swallow. Pain is experienced in this joint due to wear and tear; stress that expresses itself in grinding or clenching the teeth; misalignment of the upper and lower jaws; and, sometimes, arthritis. So spend some time massaging and relaxing this joint. It's often overlooked, but can really use whatever TLC you're willing to give it.
- With your thumb and forefinger, gently pinch the skin along the jawbone and under the chin.
- Finish by applying gentle pressure to the temples. You can also use what is called tapotement, lightly tapping your entire face with your index and middle fingers on both hands, moving from center of face outward.

Your facial muscles should now be relaxed, and you are now ready to do more deep work on scar tissue if you choose to. (Also, the above bullet points are used only as a basic guideline for your facial massage.) Feel free to incorporate anything else you have discovered that helps your face to relax.

One thing people ask me about quite frequently is if they should use some kind of massage tools. I don't personally use them very much in my practice, but as mentioned before, with using a pin or pen to sense nerve sensation, sometimes extra tools can be useful. If you want to use a tool when massaging yourself, you can try one of those loofah mitts, or any other glove made from natural fibers. These tools are good for feeling rejuvenated, and not just for facial massage. *(For example, there is a technique called body brushing which is simply a very fast brushing of the skin. Most people report feeling dramatically more awake and alert after this type of '5 minute pick me up', with a quick body brushing massage. Personally, I think work places would do well to incorporate this into their daily routine, but it might be an odd thing for all employees to take part in, which is probably why American corporations don't do it. But here's a quick overview of body brushing: You can begin with your legs, gently brushing your skin in a circular motion. You then work upward, across the thighs, towards the stomach, and in towards the heart, very quickly working in quick movements all over the body. For more information, do a Google search on body brushing.)*

Working on scar tissue in the face:

For the scar tissue itself, use a lot of facial stretches. Again, do a google search for face stretches.

Also, directly on the scar tissue, use the pinch method (incorporating skin rolling), the point/prick method, effleurage, and petrissage. Many scars on the face are directly across the face, and the skin can become pulled very tightly. If you can't get a hold of the scar tissue initially, try massaging around the scar to get it to loosen up. If you do this every day for a week or two, you should be able to get the scar to where you can do some skin rolling with it.

Having someone else work with you who is patient and understanding can also be a very healing experience when it comes to working with facial scar tissue.

Abdominals

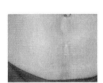 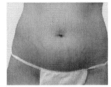

Of all the areas that people isolate as specific parts of their bodies, the stomach seems, for most people, to be one of the most sensitive.

Body metaphorics (the field of study which relates a part of the body to issues we deal with in our daily lives) says that the stomach deals with issues that get us frustrated, happy ("I felt like I had butterflies in my stomach"), nervous ("I felt so scared, I thought I was going to puke"), and most of the other emotions. Thinking about this in a general sense, the stomach relates to issues of intellect, thought, criticism, openness, orientation, and elimination.

Now if you have scar tissue of the stomach, I'm not necessarily saying that this is why you have it. But if any of these issues relate to you, they are worth thinking about, and letting go of.

To massage the stomach, you want to move in a circular motion. You will want to work on the abdomen, moving your hands clockwise, and beginning below the ribs.

 Why do I move clockwise?

Because that is the direction of peristalsis. Peristalsis is the digestive process that happens any time you eat or drink anything. If you work in a counter-clockwise motion on the stomach, you can actually cause things to 'back-up' potentially causing cramps, indigestion, and constipation.

If you're having a problem with a loose bowel, you may want to 'back things up'. (Massage can do this, but otherwise,) You will want to work clockwise, in the direction of peristalsis.

I think that the Straight Dope explains this pretty well:

"Peristalsis works just like [squeezing a tube of] toothpaste, to wit: circular and longitudinal muscles along the walls of the pharynx (throat), esophagus, stomach, and intestines contract in waves, pushing the food or whatever ahead [...] So powerful is the force created by these muscles that food passing through the pharynx is rammed down the line at a speed of about 25 feet per second. Things slow down a tad in the esophagus--here, four to eight inches of muscle contract at a time, and about nine seconds are required for the whole trip from throat to stomach."

"Gravity is a secondary consideration, coming into play only when liquids are involved. When you're sitting up, liquids drop straight through the esophagus, then wait nine seconds or so for the peristaltic contractions to catch up and open the gateway to the stomach. If you're standing on your head or bending over, peristalsis does the job just fine, as any giraffe will be happy to attest."

"Humanity has been sadly shortchanged in the peristalsis department. Cows and other cud-chewing animals (ruminants) have the ability to reverse the direction of peristalsis when necessary,(15) bringing food up from the stomach to the mouth for a few extra chomps."

 So how should I do a general stomach massage for myself?

Well, this is one of those areas that can be difficult to work on yourself. One thing that you can do for yourself is to simply rub your belly (as in pat your head while rubbing your belly). Be sure to go in the direction of peristalsis. For specific areas of scar tissue, use the pinch method (incorporating skin rolling), the point/prick method, effleurage, and petrissage. If you have areas that are hper-sensitive to touch, or not sensitive at all, be sure to use the point/prick method quite extensively.

 What can someone else do for me with a stomach massage?

If you are uncomfortable showing your breasts, they can be covered with a towel, pillowcase, or small sheet. Then, the person can begin by putting a small amount of lotion or oil on your stomach and on their hands. (As always, a good hand washing is a good idea before massage.) Lightly placing their palm on your belly button, and then lightly rolling their hand around (in a clockwise direction), have flip their hand in a rolling motion. This will be they go from having their palm on your stomach, to having the back of their hand on your stomach, and back again. This may initially feel uncomfortable as the receiver, but as you receive more stomach massage, it becomes more natural and comfortable to have this kind of work done. Most importantly, this work is not designed to be painful, so if it is, you will want to communicate with the person giving you the massage to lighten up with the pressure.

Next, they can start on the right side of your body, placing middle and pointer finger together, and placing them a centimeter or two up ('up' meaning towards your head) from the hip. Then they take their fingers, run them up to the lowest rib, across your stomach, to the lowest rib on the other side of the stomach, and run their fingers down to just above the pelvis (hip bone) on your left side. They can do this as many times as you like and as slow or as fast as you like.

They can also do what I like to call the doggie paddle pull. With this move, they reach their hands across your body. Their hands move over your side and their fingertips slide underneath your back. (Make sure they are using enough lotion or oil to not get caught on the skin.) Then have them pull, one hand at a time, up on the side. You will really feel this stretch and open up the muscles in the sides of your abdomen, and even in your back. They alternate hands, kind of like paddling, back and forth, and pulling up on your side. After they have done this on one side, they go to the other side of your body, reach across your body, and start the same on the other side.

They can then finish off by doing the squish. The Squish is fun, but it's not designed to squish anything, so don't have the person use so much pressure that you feel squishing going on internally. Standing or kneeling by your side, they put one hand across your body (on the other side of your body - kind of like they're getting ready to doggie paddle pull), and the other hand rests on the other side of your body, and then the hands lightly squish the sides of your stomach, as the hands slide towards the middle of your body and trade sides with each other. Work up and down the stomach with this move.

This type of massage, when done consistently over time, can help reduce the appearance of stretch marks resulting from pregnancy or weight loss.

If there is a specific area of scar tissue, such as from a caesarean section or other stomach surgery, the individual working with you can also use the pinch and skin rolling methods to loosen up the solid tissue formations in and around the scar tissue.

Back to sheet stretches! This move requires you to work with a partner. You lay face down. Now, if you think about it, few people could lift the middle of someone else's body without the use of the sheet, and the great thing about this move is that allows the receiver to have a really cool and unique feeling. Fold the sheet so that it's about one-foot wide. Lay so that the sheet is centered beneath your hips. Now, have the person stand on either side of your body, with their feet at about the level of your thighs, and face your head. Have the person pull the sheet up until it tugs lightly against your stomach. They really should have a good grip on the sheet, and be bending their knees slightly. Now, you take a deep breath in, and when you let the breath out, your partner lifts up on the sheet by straightening their legs and pulling up. Have them jiggle the sheet up and down, and side to side, by moving their arms. Then have them slowly lower you back to the ground. One important thing to know is that you shouldn't do this to someone who is pregnant, or if the person receiving has a problem with his or her bladder or hips.

One thing that can also help with scar tissue in the stomach, if they're not too painful (in the scar tissue) to do, are good old fashioned stomach crunches.

 I was afraid you might say that.

Hey, Don't Touch Me! Page 52

Uterine

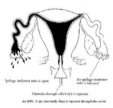

Author's Note: If this makes you uncomfortable, just skip this section of the book.

To be honest, I have no practicing knowledge of actually performing massage in this area of the body. I do know that it can become scarred emotionally, as well as physically. These scars can lead to problems with fertility, sexual frustration, and infections/diseases of the female anatomy. For this portion of the book, I have excerpt massage techniques from tantra.org, because from the little knowledge I have in this arena. I think the Yoni massage comes closest to offering a healing massage for this area of the body... If you are really interested in researching this kind of massage, and finding out how it might be able to help you or someone you know, this book will not be a comprehensive guide. I would recommend reading the techniques offered here, and then check out clearpassage.com, as well as tantra.org. They would be good starting points for further research.

As I mentioned earlier, if this makes you uncomfortable, just skip this section of the book.

Part of the uterine lining is shed each month during the menstrual cycle. Stomach & uterus corrective massage can reduce abdominal pains and distinguish healthy ovaries. Because stomach & uterus corrective massage can detect kidney malfunction and inflammation of the pancreas, it can prevent urinary tract and gallbladder disorders. It can also remove cellulite and fibrous tissues in the stomach, and you can build a healthy, strong and firm stomach through regular corrective massaging and exercising.

Dr. Arvigo is a healer and doctor trained in various approaches to health and wellness. Arvigo has become well known since the publication in 1994 of her book, *Sastun: My Apprenticeship with a Maya Healer*. This biographical story chronicles the path that led Arvigo and her husband and family to the Central American rainforest of western Belize, where she has lived and worked for almost twenty years. Dr. Arvigo's professional background is in Naprapathy, a system of therapeutic bodywork that is an offshoot of chiropractic. She graduated in 1981 from the Chicago National College of Naprapathy.

"In at least 10 percent of her practice in uterine massage over the years, she has found that women experience an emotional release during the massage process due to possible negative past experiences related to sexuality and reproduction. The treatment can, at the very least, bring tears and in more extreme cases may result in major emotional breakdowns, or "breakthroughs," that can be profound and even disturbing. Past incidents of rape, incest, traumatic childbirth, abortions, infertility and so forth can evoke emotions that have been in the tissues and muscles of the pelvis and may be spontaneously released when deep massage is done by a trusted practitioner whose purpose is to heal[…]

"Arvigo likened this phenomenon of releasing emotional and psychic armor to the muscular armor rings described by the famous psychoanalyst Wilhelm Reich in the 1930s. Arvigo describes Reich as the "father of bodywork" and urged participants to read his classic work on the subject in *Character Analysis*. In his work, Reich identified seven different areas or bands in the body where different kinds of emotions and trauma were held in, and then eventually were manifest as physical symptoms or disease in that area.

"Arvigo stated that [Reich's] "seventh muscular armor ring," centered in the pelvis and genitals, is precisely the area where uterine massage evokes the same shame and guilt and subsequent pain described by Reich decades ago.

"Arvigo warned that if the emotional breakthroughs are a result of significant prior physical or emotional trauma, it may be necessary to refer the individual for intensive counseling and/or psychoanalytic work in addition to treatment with uterine massage techniques." [11]

Background Information on Yoni Massage:

(The rest of this section is used with permission from http://www.tantra.org/yoni.html)

Yoni (pronounced YO-NEE) is a Sanskrit word for the female reproductive system that is loosely translated as "Sacred Space" or "Sacred Temple." Its meaning and use is an alternate perspective from the Western view of the female genitals. In Tantra, the Yoni is seen from a perspective of love and respect. This is especially helpful for men to learn.

The purpose of the Yoni Massage is to create a space for the woman (the receiver) to relax, and enter a state of high arousal and experience much pleasure from her Yoni. Her partner (the giver) experiences the joy of being of service and witnessing a special moment. The Yoni Massage can also be used as a form of safer sex (when latex gloves are used) and is an excellent activity to build trust and intimacy. Some massage and sex therapists use it to assist women to break through sexual blocks or trauma.

The goal of the Yoni massage is not orgasm. Orgasm is often a pleasant and welcome side effect. The goal is simply to pleasure and massage the Yoni.

From this perspective both receiver and giver can relax, and not have to worry about achieving something. When orgasm does occur it is usually more expanded, more intense and more satisfying. Orgasm is allowed to happen or not happen. It is also helpful for the giver to not expect anything in return. Just allow the receiver to enjoy the massage and to relax into herself afterwards. Of course, other sexual activity may follow but it should be entirely the receiver's choice.
This perspective will build greater intimacy and trust, and will greatly expand your sexual horizons.

PREPARATION: Bathing is always helpful as it relaxes both the receiver and giver. A quiet space is desirable with pleasing music, candles, pillows, etc., or whatever makes the participants relax and feel safe. Allow yourself enough time and do not hurry through the process. Go to the bathroom before beginning the massage. The best results will occur when the bowels and bladder are empty and you will avoid the unnecessary experience of interrupting the massage to go to the bathroom. Connect with your partner by hugging, holding, eye gazing (looking into each other's eyes for an extended time), or whatever brings you to a place of safety and relaxation.

PROCEDURE: Have the receiver lie on her back with pillows under her head so she can look down at herself and up at her partner (giver). Place a pillow, covered with a towel, under her hips. Her legs are to be spread apart with the knees slightly bent (pillows or cushions under the knees will also help)[…] The giver sits cross-legged between the receivers' legs. The giver may wish to sit on a pillow or cushion. This position allows full access to the Yoni and other parts of the body. Before contacting the body, begin with deep, relaxed breathing. Both giver and receiver should remember to keep breathing deeply, slowly and with relaxation during the entire process. The giver will gently remind the receiver to start breathing again if the receiver stops or takes shallower breaths. Deep breathing, not hyperventilating, is very important here.

Gently massage the legs, abdomen, thighs, breasts, etc., to get the receiver to relax and for the giver to prepare for touching the Yoni. Pour a small quantity of a high-quality oil or lubricant on the mound of the Yoni. Pour just enough so that it drips down the outer lips and covers the outside of the Yoni. (Several excellent sexual lubricants are available for this. Many lingerie shops, sex toy shops, sex magazines, etc., offer these safe lubricants.)

CAVEAT - Do not mix oil-based products with latex.

Begin gently massaging the mound and outer lips of the Yoni. Spend some time here and do not rush. Relax and enjoy giving the massage. Gently squeeze the outer lip between the thumb and index finger, and slide up and down the entire length of each lip. Do the same thing to the inner lips of the Yoni. Take your time.

The receiver can massage her own breasts or may just relax and continue breathing deeply. It is helpful for giver and receiver to look into each other's eyes as much as possible. The receiver can tell the giver if the pressure, speed, depth, etc., needs to be increased or decreased. Limit your speaking and focus on the pleasurable sensations[…].

Gently stroke the clitoris with clockwise and counter-clockwise circles. Gently squeeze it between thumb and index fingers. Do this as a massage and not to [have the receiver be sexually aroused]. The receiver will undoubtedly become very aroused but continue to encourage her to just relax and breathe.

Slowly and with great care, insert the middle finger of your right hand into the Yoni (there is a reason for using the right hand as opposed to the left. It has to do with polarity in Tantra). Very gently explore and massage the inside of the Yoni with this finger. Take your time, be gentle, and feel up, down and sideways. Vary the depth, speed and pressure. Remember, this is a massage and you're nurturing and relaxing the Yoni. With your palm facing up, and the middle finger inside the Yoni, move the middle finger in a "come here" gesture or crook back towards the palm. You will contact a spongy area of tissue just under the pubic bone, behind the clitoris. This is the "G-spot" or in Tantra, the sacred spot [The receiver] may feel as if they have to urinate or it may be painful or pleasurable. Again vary the pressure, speed and pattern of movement. You can move side to side, back and forth, or in circles with your middle finger. You can also insert the finger that's between your middle finger and pinky. Check with your partner [before using two fingers] […]Take your time and be very gentle. You may use the thumb of the right hand to stimulate the clitoris as well[…].

So, what is your left hand doing all this time? You can use it to massage the breasts, abdomen, or clitoris. If you massage the clitoris it's usually best to use your thumb in an up down motion, with the rest of your hand resting on and massaging the mound. The dual stimulation of right and left hands will provide much pleasure for the receiver. I do not recommend using your left hand to touch your own genitals because it may take your focus off the receiver. Remember, this massage is for her pleasure and much of the benefit comes from not only the physical stimulation but the intent as well. Continue massaging, trying different speeds, pressures and motions[…] She may have powerful emotions come up and may cry. Just keep breathing and be gentle. Many women have been sexually abused and need to be healed. A giving, loving and patient partner can be of great value to her.

Breast

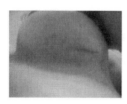 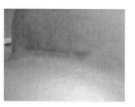

This is another section that could make you uncomfortable. If this makes you uncomfortable, just skip this section of the book.

Breast massage helps to increase the circulation in your breasts and decreases the symptoms of PMS, menopause and menstrual cramps. Therapeutic breast massage can also lessen discomforts associated with breast cancer treatments, help relieve post-surgical symptoms, and reduce discomfort from pregnancy, breastfeeding and weaning. Breast massage also contributes to improved skin tone while promoting relaxation and balancing your energy.

Regular breast massage, either done by yourself, or done by someone else, has the positive benefits of regular massage mentioned elsewhere in this book. One of the challenges with the breasts, however, which make them different from other parts of the body, are that many women and men get to where they feel uncomfortable with this area of their bodies, and as a result, exercise a daily pattern of neglect. This pattern, when practiced over years, leads to blockages in the breast tissue, the lymph nodes, and the muscles in the area.

With regular massage, you will help diminish benign breast cysts while helping to flush lymph nodes and stimulating your glandular system. The breasts are soft tissue and do not have muscles to help them move.

Breasts can be effectively self-massaged or massaged by a professional massage therapist. Gentle hands-on techniques, with breast either uncovered or lightly draped, will help enhance circulation and drainage. It's important to understand the anatomy of the breast before doing work on it.

"Each breast contains 15 to 20 lobes arranged in a circular fashion. The fat (subcutaneous adipose tissue) that covers the lobes gives the breast its size and shape. Each lobe is comprised of many lobules, at the end of which are tiny bulb like glands, or sacs, where milk is produced in response to hormonal signals.

"Ducts connect the lobes, lobules, and glands in nursing mothers. These ducts deliver milk to openings in the nipple. The areola is the darker-pigmented area around the nipple. (16)

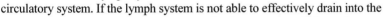

In breast massage, the areas that are focused on are the muscle tissue, the skin, and the lymph nodes. Lymph nodes hold toxins, because it is the primary job of the lymph system to remove toxins. The lymph system ties into the circulatory system. If the lymph system is not able to effectively drain into the circulatory system, (this can be caused by inactivity or lack of touch) then the toxins can become bound up in the lymph and muscular systems, which can lead to problems with breastfeeding, disease, and, arguably, can even lead to cancer.

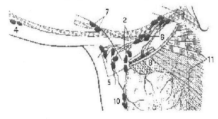

Now that you have a better understanding of how the breast tissue is laid out, and what all is involved in the breast, it is important that you use the knowledge to your benefit. People say that knowledge equals power. This is only partially true. Knowledge + activity = the ability to gain more knowledge = power. That thought included, the four-step procedure that is talked about in this book is a simple massage technique that can be done by yourself. Although almost any gentle massage technique will benefit the various systems involved in the breast tissue, these four techniques from BodyMechanics.net should be part of what you do on a weekly, if not daily, basis.

The purpose doing these things is to create movement in the breast tissue, flushing out old fluids from the breast, (both in the veins and in between the cells), and bringing in nutrients and oxygen. Also, using this sort of a massage on a regular basis helps to enhance the health and elasticity of the ligaments supporting the breast, which will give you better breast support. You can do these techniques for yourself, or if you feel comfortable, have a partner do them with/for you.

From BodyMechanics.net:

"More specifically, step one is a gentle draining motion designed to drain the breast's lymphatic system, and is possibly the most important of the four steps. Steps number[s] two and four are to assist in the movement of venous fluids. Feel free to experiment with these to movements and find what is comfortable for you. Step three is simply to help keep your support ligaments in good health and assist in the fight against gravity.

This procedure should be done at least twice a week. It can be done on bare skin, but you may find that using some vegetable oil may be more comfortable. Stay away from mineral-based or scented oils.

 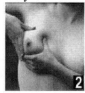 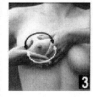 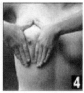

Step One: Use your fingers to gently smooth away from the nipple. These movements travel from the nipple and directly away using no more pressure than what you would apply to your eyelid. Any more pressure would flatten the lymphatic vessel and stop the flow of toxins and fluids. Also, make this stroke slow, not fast, for it to be effective.

Step Two: Gently massage the breast with a kneading-like motion, using lifting and pressing movements.

Step Three: Slowly and carefully use your hands to twist the breast in a clock-wise and counterclockwise direction, being careful not to put too much tension on the breast.

Step Four: Use both hands as shown to apply several compressions, using moderate pressure, to move out more pressure fluids."

Stretching the muscles around the breast tissue will be important in relaxing the breast itself. Try doing Google searches to find stretches for the following muscles:

Pectoralis Stretches   Oblique stretches   Anterior serratus stretches

Back

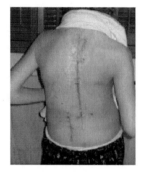

Just how bad can a bad back be? Back pain is the worst, according to sufferers of chronic (ongoing) back pain.

Maybe you're one of the people who has chronic back pain. If you are, I really highly recommend a few things:
- Have a doctor take a look at you to see what is going on.
- Work with massage therapists who help you feel emotionally comforted, and who are willing to help you work through the deeper tissue (using Neuro-Muscular Techniques), at a pressure level that is uncomfortable, but not painful, for you).
- Use surgery only as a LAST, LAST, LAST, LAST, LAST (did I say that enough times?) LAST resort. Try everything else before having back surgery. I have never known anyone who was 100% happy with their back surgery, or the results that they had after it.

Maybe you've already had back surgery, and maybe you're okay with the results, but you are wondering how to diminish the scarring effects in your back. If that's the case, this is the right place for you to be looking.

The back is very complex, because of the variety of muscles, the directions they run, and the actions that the back can do. So, rather than spending a lot of time on the anatomy of the back, I would like to give you some simple exercises that can be done for yourself, and also, give you some massage, that someone else can do for you.

What you can do for yourself:

Well, to be honest, it can be quite difficult to do your own back massage (and I would argue that it's relatively impossible to give yourself back massage). So your ability to work with scar tissue in your back is going to be limited to your patience with visualizing what is going on in your body, and to stretching.

But, you can use Ed Moore's Do-It-Yourself Tennis Ball Back Massage. Ed Moore is a certified massage therapist who has worked with the U.S. Olympic cycling team.

So, before you start, you can slide two tennis balls into a sock (or racquetballs, although tennis balls work better), tying off the open end of the sock so that the tennis balls are touching each other.

What you will want to do is take a hot bath or shower, to loosen the muscles, followed by some gentle stretching, also to loosen the muscles of the back. Next, you will lie on your back on the floor or another flat surface... although a carpeted surface tends to be best for most people. Have the sock nearby, and place it under your back, making sure that one ball sits on each side of your spine.

Take a deep breath in, and as you let it out, let your body relax down on the tennis balls. This will probably be uncomfortable, but shouldn't cause a lot of pain. From here, you can do a lot of movements. Rock your hips gently from side to side, or up and down. Then adjust your body so that the sock and tennis balls move up your back a few inches. Hold that position briefly, and then breathe deeply. You should start to feel your back muscles kind of loosening up to the pressure of the tennis balls, and when you feel this (may take up to 30 seconds), then you can move the sock and tennis balls further up your back.

Take a minimum of 5 minutes to work the tennis balls up and down your back, but if you have a particularly sore area, spend extra time with the tennis balls under that spot in your back, and rock your hips up and down, as well as side to side, until you feel your body relax into the tennis balls. So there you have it, at least one unique movement you can do for your own back.

Having someone else work on your back can be done in a variety of ways. This book isn't designed to be a book on massage basics, but there is something really great and relaxing about getting a back massage. This relaxation can help the tissues all over your body (not just in your back) open up, which is why I have included instructions for a basic back massage in this book. I actually am fortunate in that BodyMechanics allowed me to use their back massage technique for this book, so, without further ado, here it is:

"Most people massage their friend's back while they lie on the floor or on a bed. We [Body Mechanics] suggest that they lay on the floor on top of a series of couch cushions or futon type cushion. Position yourself on your knees beside them. Use your weight and be careful not to strain your own back. For optimum access to their back, it will be helpful to have them remove their shirt and to pull their underwear down a bit. Be sure to have them turn their head occasionally so their neck won't get stiff."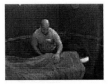

"Before we begin, it is important to note the areas that can be accidentally injured with too much pressure. These areas are marked in red in the photo [...]. The lower two red spots are the approximate locations of the kidneys. Never do percussive (pounding) techniques here. Secondly, don't dig deep into the armpits without additional training. Also be careful of the sciatic nerve in the buttocks.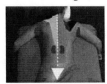
Sharp pressure in this area will be very painful. Also, note the white dots on the photo above. These dots indicate the approximate location of the bones called the spinous processes. Don't press directly on these bones. Don't push on these bones with pressure thinking that they are just [knots or other bumps. They're actually bones!]."

Now on to the actual back massage. Again, remember that you should feel free to try your own techniques; this is just provided as a very beginner's guide to getting the back muscles to relax through massage.

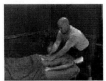
From the head (top) smooth down the back muscles on both sides of the spine. This thick rope-like muscle is called the Erector Spinae group. It actually runs from the base of the skull to the tail bone area. Use equal pressure on your fingers and the heels of your hands. Smooth down the Erector Spinae, and back up along your friend's sides, shoulders, and neck. Do this several times. Move yourself along their side

and face their head. Repeat the long smoothing strokes, going slightly deeper
with each pass. Make sure that your hands conform
to their body. Your pressure should be even and
your strokes consistent in speed. Try splitting your
index finger and your center finger, placing your
hand over the spine. Gently place each finger in the
groove between the spine and the Erector Spinae
muscles[…]."

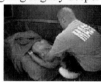

"We will now work the side. Begin working the
buttocks area by" [*I'm going to interrupt here and
offer a different Gluteus Maximus massage
technique, because I like it better. Do what we call
"Kitty Paws". Kitty paws are simply forming fists*

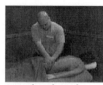

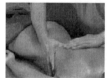

*with your hands and gently pushing into the gluteal
muscles, alternating left and right hands, kind of like a
kitty paws at a, well, anything,… only be more fluid
and gentle with your movements
than a kitty would be. That's it.
It's pretty easy.*] "Continue up
the back by lifting and scooping the sides, alternating
hands. Make sure that your movements are confident and
firm, so that you don't tickle your friend. As you
get to the top of the shoulders, lift and scoop the thick muscle, known as the
upper Trapezius, as shown in the picture[…]."

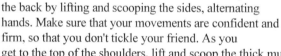
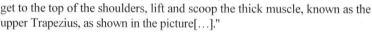

"As your scooping strokes return back down the side, try lifting the shoulder
gently off of the table and letting it gently slip through
your fingers as the weight pulls it
back to the floor. Now, place one
hand over the sacrum (you
might call it the tail bone) as
shown to the right, and begin
rocking it, with pressure, to the left and right […].
Follow up with your thumbs making strokes up and away from the sacrum
area. Gently work the whole area."

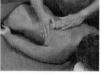
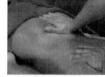

Hey, Don't Touch Me! Page 64

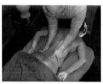"Again begin making strokes down the back, but deeper than the first time. Emphasize your pressure on the heel of your hands, stroking the Erector Spinae, down both sides of the spine. You can try to separate the fibers of the Erector Spinae group of muscles with your thumb. For extra strength, you can use your other fingers to reinforce your thumb. Firmly, but smoothly, work from the ditch next to the spine and over the Erector Spinae muscle. Don't "thump" over the muscle. Take it slowly, with 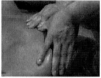 control. This will help to improve the fibers in the muscle itself."

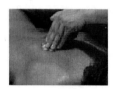"After you've worked the muscle all the way down the back, you can do soothing circular strokes with the finger tips along the same area. This serves to relax the muscle and increase circulation."

As I've said, this book isn't designed to be an instruction book on how to give massage, but rather an overview for getting the muscles to relax, which will aid dramatically in scar tissue healing. For more information on how to give an in-depth back massage, visit Bodymechanics.net.

For more information on back stretches, check out Google searches for the following muscle stretches

Levator stretches
Latissimus dorsi stretches
Trapezius stretches
Spinal Erector stretches
Quadratus Lumborum stretches

One thing that someone else can do for you is…

 Sheet stretches?

Yes, you got it!!!

Hey, Don't Touch Me! Page 65

This is very much like the stomach sheet stretch. What it does is open up the lower and middle back, encouraging the spine to adjust itself.

Lay face up on the floor. Fold the sheet to form a two-foot-wide panel. Place the sheet underneath your hips. Have the person who is working with you place one foot on each side of you, facing your head. They will lightly but firmly pull the sheet snug up against your buttocks and lower back. They should bend their knees while you take a big breath. When you let your breath out, the person working with you will straighten their knees, lift up on the sheet, and lean back. This will raise the middle of your torso slightly off the ground. Now you should hold this for a few seconds, and then they slowly lower your body to the ground or surface you're on. They will wait for a minute, allowing you to feel your body on the ground once again. Then, they will lift again. This time though, have them alternate moving their arms up and down so that you are being lifted on one side of your back, and then the other - kind of like you are being rocked side to side.

A couple things to be aware of - don't do this on someone with back problems. It also should not be attempted on someone whose weight you cannot easily manage.

Shoulders

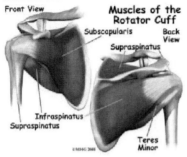
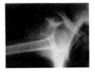

Shoulders, like knees, are quite complex, and one of the most used (and abused,) joints in the body. As a result, shoulder surgeries are common, and these surgeries can result in scarring in many places within the shoulder, as well as in the muscle tissue and in the more superficial (outer) layers of the skin.

As we talk about the shoulder, I want you to think about this guy. Many people think that their shoulder pain is bad, and they often get into a mindset of "I am the only person in the world who really understands what it's like to be me. No 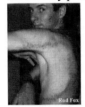 one else can possibly understand my pain!" This may not be you, but you may know someone, who has that kind of thinking. The next time you think that, think about this guy. See the marks all the way around his armpit, in a half-circle? Kind of almost like a big mouth sucked on his side? Well, a big mouth BIT his side.
This gentleman spent three years recovering from a shark bite (yes, a shark bit this part of his body) which nearly cost him not only his arm or shoulder, but his life.

If he can rehab from a bite this bad, (shark's teeth were stuck in his shoulder when the shark finally let go) you can definitely rehabilitate your shoulder from whatever you're going through!

If you have shoulder pain, you should see a doctor to get their opinion. Your doctor's first goal will be to control as much of the pain and inflammation as possible. Initial treatment is likely to be rest and anti-inflammatory medication, such as aspirin or ibuprofen. The anti-inflammatory medicine is used mainly to control pain. Your doctor may suggest a cortisone injection if you have trouble getting your pain under control. Cortisone is a strong anti-inflammatory, and I recommend people against it. It's not just my opinion either.

In *My Top Ten Reasons Not to Get A Cortisone Shot*, Ross A. Hauser, M.D., offers many reasons not to have cortisone injected into your joints. I particularly thought this one summed it up well:

" Reason #9: Cortisone Shots Keep People From Getting Healing Therapies

"People want the easy way out. We have instant oatmeal, drive-up lunch stops, drive-up espresso, soon we will have drive-up bathrooms. Don't ask me how the latter will work.

"What is easier than getting a cortisone shot? "Why not? Insurance will pick it up." Yeah, right buddy, they will pick up your future hip replacement too!

"By getting a cortisone shot and masking the pain, people do not get the healing therapies they need. Any therapy that helps increase circulation to the area helps healing. Therapies such as exercise, myofascial release, rolfing, magnets, massage, chiropractic physiotherapy, kinesiotherapy, acupuncture, herbs, vitamins, and a host of others help people truly heal injuries. When people pop anti-inflammatories and get cortisone shots - it is like taking the battery out of a blaring fire alarm while a fire is blazing. "No problem here!" "What do you mean, you dope! The alarm means there's a fire!" This illustration seems silly. Who would take the batteries out of the fire alarm during a blazing fire and state "no problem here."

"Yeah, stupid, huh? Well, what could be stupider than have a fire blazing in a tendon, ligament, or joint and stomping out the healing with a cortisone shot? Don't take the "alarm signalers" out of your injured structures." [17]

So outside of the cortisone discussion, here's what you can do to reduce the scar tissue in your shoulder.

What you can do for yourself:
The shoulder can be difficult to work on by yourself, similar to the back. But, for the skin and muscles you can effectively reach with the opposite hand, try using the pinch method (of course using skin rolling), the point/prick method, effleurage, and petrissage.

You can also do stretching for the shoulder. You can find some good stretches to isolate the different muscles which tie into the shoulder by doing Google searches for stretches for the following muscles.

subscapularis stretch
teres minor stretch
pectoralis minor stretch
upper trapezius stretch

infraspinatus stretch
supraspinatus stretch
pectoralis major stretch

What someone else can do for you:
Techniques that encourage relaxation of the muscles surrounding the shoulder are where basic shoulder massage should focus. Simple techniques, such as effleurage and broad cross-fiber sweeping strokes are useful in the shoulder. What can happen in the shoulder, due to the limited range of motion in the shoulder, is that the muscles can become kind of fibery (as in, isolated into individual fibers, rather than being a muscle group), and they can also become shorter. The goal of shoulder massage, and especially more advanced shoulder massage, is to get the full range of movement back into the shoulder.

What I've provided here is simply a basic shoulder and neck massage which can be done by anyone to help the muscles in and around the shoulder to relax, reduce muscle tension, and also reduce the stress which can be associated with shoulder injuries and scar tissue.

Use these steps to give your friend a shoulder and neck massage.

1. Have your friend sit straight but comfortably in a chair. Place your hands on your friend's shoulders.
2. Knead the two muscles on either side of the neck next to the shoulders. Start with very little pressure, then squeeze harder.
3. Work on the back of the neck.
    - Have your friend lean his or her head forward.
    - Support your friend's forehead firmly with one of your hands. This lets your friend's neck muscles relax.
    - With the thumb and first finger of your other hand, make tiny circles at the base of the skull.
    - Gently squeeze the entire back of the neck. Bring your friend's head up to its normal position.
4. Use a "thumb crawling" technique.
    - Press both thumbs down, one on the outside of each shoulder.
    - Move them in, pressing firmly at intervals of 0.5 in.(1.27 cm) until both thumbs reach the spine at the same time.
    - "Crawl" your thumbs out again to the shoulder joints.

- Repeat this movement 4 or 5 times.
5. With one hand on each shoulder, knead the upper back and shoulders. Work your hands away from each other, ending at the upper arms. Then reverse the process by massaging back to either side of the neck. [18]

Sort of as an aside: If your therapy program doesn't stabilize your shoulder after a period of time, you may decide to have surgery. Just remember that surgery will lead to scar tissue, which will need to be worked through. There are many different types of shoulder operations to stabilize the shoulder. Almost all of these operations attempt to tighten the ligaments that are loose. The loose ligaments are usually along the front or bottom part of the shoulder capsule. With some time and consistency, massage and/or physical therapy can generally achieve the same results as these surgeries, unless the injury to the shoulder is such that the ligaments or tendons have torn away from the bones. If that's the case (where the attachments have torn away from the bones), then surgery is often necessary and effective.

The most common method for surgically stabilizing a shoulder that is prone to anterior dislocations is the Bankart repair. The Bankart repair involves sewing or stapling ligaments on the front side of the joint back into their original position. First, the doctor clears away any frayed or torn edges. Holes for the sutures are drilled into the scapula bone. The capsular ligaments are then attached with sutures to the bone.

The ligaments heal, and scar tissue eventually anchors the ends to the bone. With the ligaments back in place, the joint is [generally] much more stable.

Typically the Bankart repair is done through an incision on the front of the shoulder. Some doctors prefer to perform a similar operation using an arthroscope. This new technique is not yet widely practiced. Arthroscopes require smaller incisions, which means less time in the hospital and less time to heal. [19]

The point of all this is, your doctor may be someone who likes to use surgery as a frequent solution to all problems, or your doctor may only use surgery as a last resort. I highly recommend having massage therapy and physical therapy at least 6 months before having shoulder surgery. I would recommend at least bi-monthly (twice per month) trips to the massage therapist and physical therapist, but if you can go once per week, you will probably notice results more quickly.

Feet

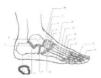 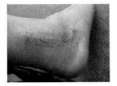

According medical studies conducted in China, as far back as 2000 years ago, massage of the reflex zones in the feet and hands can cause changes in the relative nerves elsewhere in the body. Chinese medicine works to relax those nerves, because doing so and can promote better blood circulation. The logic of 2000 years ago went on to say that the increased blood circulation will affect a person's health condition, because circulation is vital to every organ.

Where did we go wrong in Western medicine? (*Do you feel the soapbox coming out? Please allow me to stand on it for just a minute.*) I mean, don't get me wrong here, because there are great things about western medicine, but there are some very simple things that western medicine often overlooks.

Blood is the medium for the transport of nutrients, oxygen, hormones, antibodies, amino acids, structural proteins, cells, and waste. What that means is that the better the circulation is, the healthier the individual body will be. It is simple logic, and it works. The U. S. spends billions more on healthcare than China, for a large variety of reasons, including the approach they take to healthcare in China. Some say China's healthcare is less adequate than the U.S., but this is arguable. China also serves a much larger population of people than the U.S., so there has to be something to how they keep their healthcare costs significantly lower. Might it have something to do with the perspectives taught in China about the nervous system (also known as your reflexes)?

An unbalanced nervous system can cause insomnia, heart arrhythmia, constipation, tiredness, migraine, and aches and pains, for reasons which both Chinese and western medicine have yet to fully explain. However, these imbalances can be adjusted with the right kind of reflexology massage. This can increase the health of your nerve reflexes, relax nervous muscles, and calm the pain of tired and sore nerves.

I will be sharing with you here how you can so some simple foot massage and exercises in the feet and hands to promote healing in the rest of the body. *(We won't be delving too much into reflexology, because it's really a book on its own, and the purpose of this book is to give you some simple ways to relax the tissues around the scar tissue, and to work with the scar tissue itself. Some reflexology will happen naturally, simply by massaging the soles of the feet, while mentally focusing on tender places, but the massage offered here is more of a general guideline for helping your feet to feel great!)*

Learning to give a good foot massage is one of the nicest gifts you can give to your own two feet, or to those of a friend!

You should have two or three big towels on hand and some lotion, oil, or cream. A good cream works better than hand lotion or oil for the calluses and hardened skin that can form on the feet (particularly if you like to go barefoot in the summer, but any cream or lotion will work.

If you are having a friend work on you, make sure that your knee and foot are supported while your friend works on you. One good place you can use is a recliner chair with the foot rest up, with the giver either on the floor or on a small stool in front of the open foot rest.

Okay, this next point is huge! CLEAN YOUR FEET! As a massage therapist, people most often come to me having recently showered, and with good overall hygiene. But there have been times, especially working on people's feet, when I have had to pull out disinfectant hand gel just to feel okay about touching their feet. If you really want to have your feet relax, try using a foot soak with a cup of Epsom salt dissolved in a gallon of warm water. It's a great way de-stress and start loosening up the muscles before you receive a foot massage. Dry your feet thoroughly, including between your toes.

I want to offer you one quick warning about the feet. The feet have billions of tiny nerve endings in them. Some people have more nerve endings in their feet than others. These nerves can make the feet an extremely ticklish part of the body. A couple ways to overcome this are to use more of the surface of your hands (avoiding small, specific pressure), and to use more pressure. Lighter pressure on the feet can cause people to be ticklish. If someone's feet are too ticklish for you to even touch them (including your own), you might just hold the feet for a few minutes trying to relax and let the nerves come out of their heightened state of awareness.

To start, just gently rub one foot all over. Then massage the other foot. Do this just nice and relaxed. You really want to get the cream (or lotion) into the whole foot, top and bottom, toes to ankle. You can end this beginning part of the massage with some simple strokes going from the toes to the ankles.

For the next part, you will want to work with a bit more pressure. Put both hands around one foot, with your fingers on the sole and your thumbs on the top. Move your thumbs between the tendons on the top of the feet (they may feel like cords or tight small ropes). Do this smoothly and firmly from the ankle toward the toes. If you are working on someone else, make sure that this isn't painful for them, by asking "Is that too much/not enough pressure?" or "How's that pressure?"). Make long strokes on the foot for this part of the massage. Work with enough pressure so that it's not ticklish, but check in with the receiver to make sure that it's not too much pressure either. I always share with my clients that they want to have me work at a level that is uncomfortable, but not painful, because that is where the greatest amount of change will happen in their body. You want to be able to be worked with at that level, and want the people you're working with to be comfortable being worked on at that level. Don't push to get to this level though.
Sometimes it can take as many as ten sessions before people feel can be okay being worked on at an uncomfortable level.

Next, work on the soles of your feet. When you are working on yourself, this is easiest with your foot propped on the opposite knee, with a towel underneath your foot to protect your clothing from cream. Using your thumbs, make circular motions that cover the entire surface of the bottom of your foot, moving from the base of your toes toward your heel. Keep the pressure of the circles steady and even. Use a bit more firmness on your heels, even digging a knuckle into the heel if that feels appropriate. The skin and the muscle at the heel is tougher than in the rest of the foot.

If the receiver of the massage is still comfortable with the pressure, increase the pressure a bit more, and go back over the entire surface of the sole. Give a few extra strokes to any area where there is an experience of ongoing pain. These areas can include the ball of the foot, the arch, or around your ankles. One thing to remember is that you should avoid really digging in deeply, because the intention of this massage is to help the muscles relax. One way to relieve muscle cramps in the arch of the foot is to hold gentle pressure with one hand, and stretch your foot with the other, but not to the point of pain, just where it's uncomfortable, and where you're feeling muscle resistance. You can also do calf stretches to reduce cramping.

Don't forget about your toes! Use gentle, circular motions, using a bit of a stretch while you rub. Then, exercise your toes by rotating them a bit. Grip all your toes together. You can do this by placing your thumb underneath the toes, and all your fingers on top, laid crosswise across your toes. Gently rotate your toes a few times in one direction, and then reverse the direction and rotate them a few times that way. Now, let go of all the toes, and work each toe one by one… gently… but you can pull if you feel the need to "pop" your toe(s)

Shake the energy loose from your own hands if you feel it building up. This is not going to happen for all people, so if it doesn't happen for you, don't worry about it. Although excess energy tends to accumulate in the feet and be released by massage, not all people feel it, even among massage therapists, physical therapists, and other professional body workers.

You can twist the foot by rotating both hands around it. This is like when you were a kid and used to do that Indian burn thing to other kids…

 I never did that. People did that to me!

Oh… er… ummm, right. Well, that's what I meant.

Rotate your hands around the foot, each going in opposite directions. To avoid the "Indian burn" effect, use plenty of lotion or cream or oil… whatever you're using.

You can wrap up the massage in lots of different ways, but one nice thing you can to is just to repeat the all-over gentle massage you started with. Make sure you have good pressure on the foot, and work all the different parts around the ankle, between the tendons on top of the foot, between and on the pads of the toes, and on the toes themselves.

There are some people who believe that you should always move the massage strokes towards the ankles. The reason for this directional movement is that, as we age, the skin and tissue in our feet tend to migrate toward our toes, leaving our ankles bony and without proper support. That affects our balance, and there are some who say that we can help to prevent this by carefully moving things back the other direction. The jury is still out on that for me personally. However, if you feel like it will have more effects for you, feel free to use what works, and leave behind what doesn't. This isn't rocket science, and you know best what is going on your body.

After the massage, you can wipe the underside of your feet with a towel. This can help your feet to not be slippery and then you can get something cozy on your feet, like heavy cotton socks or your favorite (clean) slippers!

 What about the scar tissue in my feet? You never addressed that?

Well, I really did. If you look at these massage techniques, they are designed to help the foot, (the skin and the muscles) relax. They are also designed to improve the circulation in the foot. For working specifically on scar tissue in the feet, I recommend specifically the point/prick method, because the nerve endings in the feet are sensitive to pick up a lot of smaller sensations. These sensations, over time, will help your scar tissue redevelop nerve pathways, which will increase circulation and cut down on the thickness and the severity of the scar tissue.

Other Parts and Considerations

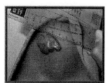

A keloid on the shoulder

"Keloids are overgrowths of scar tissue that follow injuries. Keloids may appear after such minor trauma as ear piercing. Dark skinned individuals tend to form keloids more readily than lighter skinned individuals."[10]

 What should I do about a keloid?

See a doctor. I really am in no position on what to offer you for a keloid, because generally, keloids will need to be surgically removed. If you do have to have yours surgically removed, work on the resulting scar tissue using the pinch method (incorporating skin rolling), the point/prick method, effleurage, and petrissage.

As for the rest of the body, I really struggled with this portion of the book. I know that there are parts of the body I haven't specifically covered (hands, arms, chest, neck) and I know that this will probably mean that I will get questions from people asking me how to work on parts that I haven't specifically covered.

I have set up a web page where you can ask me questions about specific scar tissue issues, so feel free to visit the page and ask me a question. Aside from that, make sure to experiment with some of the techniques offered in this book:

- point/prick
- cross-fibering
- Pinch Method/skin rolling
- Effleurage/Petrissage

These techniques will aid in the reduction and loosening of scar tissue, anywhere in the body, so long as you take the time you need to apply them.

 So is that it? Is the book over?

No silly Monkey! The book is now going to explain to you how you can take the techniques offered in this book, and apply them in your already busy life, so that you can get the maximum results, in the least amount of time possible.

 That sounds interesting and useful!

It is! Keep reading!

Part III. "Hey, I'm busy!"

How can I fit this in?

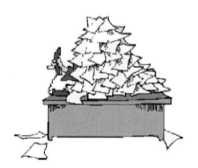

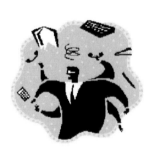

How can I fit this in?

This is a necessary and very important part of the book, because it allows you to create healing in your body, without changing your entire life and schedule.

This section of the book offers you ways to do your own healing, without restructuring your life. In other words, it gives you practical ways to incorporate the activities suggested throughout the book into what you already do.

One thing you have to realize is that your healing is already sitting in your pockets! You just don't know it yet. Please allow me to explain.

You have a 9-5, which, with the commute and headaches, has probably turned into more like a 7:30-6:30. You maybe have kids, a spouse, a dog, a car to repair, and a leaky faucet. You have yard-work, housework, homework, and work-work.

However, you understand that people do heal quickly and effectively. You think that you could heal more quickly, if only you could make it fit in your schedule. You understand some of the basic concepts of healing, and after reading this book, you more than likely understand the activities you can do to heal.

So, where will you find the time to stretch, effleurage, petrissage, do deep tissue, and use the pinch method?

The answer is in your thinking. Your thinking has to help your healing, before and while your body is healing. Then you have to live a lifestyle (in your pockets of time) that actively promotes healing in your body.

Here is what your thinking has to realize. Your healing is already in your pockets. I'll say that again. The healing is ALREADY sitting in your pockets.

How can your healing be in your pockets? Your healing is in the pockets of TIME you have. You have ten minutes here, and twenty minutes there. You have time while the pot is on the stove boiling water, and you have time while you're waiting for your kids at their soccer practice.

You have pockets of time, and if you would like to heal more effectively, and quickly, you must learn to use the pockets you do have more effectively, starting today.

(This has as much to do with planning your life as it does healing your body. If you get good at this, you can take this skill and apply it anywhere, for anything you want to accomplish.)

So how can you use your pockets effectively?

Are you ready? It's easy to do, but what's easy to do is easy not to do. Here are 5 simple steps to making healing, and being healthy, a reality!

#1. Decide

Make a decision that you are going to work on healing your body each day, no matter what. You must do some kind of activity, preferably some kind of activity outlined in this book, or another activity you've experienced positive results with. Decide that you are going to make this healing become solid within 6 months. (Be realistic with yourself. If you're only working on your healing for 15 minutes/day, then depending on the severity of the scar and the injury or trauma to the area, 6 months can be a very realistic goal.)

#2. Take action in the right direction

Begin with the end in mind. You may have heard this before, but maybe you've never applied it. Today is the time to apply it to your healing. Begin with the end in mind. For the next 5 days, take 15 minutes/day, and get your plan on paper. Figure out what you want your healthy life and healthy body look like. Look at the scar itself. How do you want it to look at 1 month, 2 months 4 months, 6 months? How do you want it to feel at 1 month, 2 months 4 months, 6 months? What will having it feel and look that way mean for your life at 1 month, 2 months 4 months, 6 months?

Put your goals on paper. Have friends (and even strangers if you like) review your plans. Ask for their honest feedback. Don't be offended if they tell you that you might try being more realistic. Also don't be offended if they tell you that you can achieve more than what you have on paper. You can do whatever you decide to do, as long as it's SMART. Having it on paper will help you. Take what works and leave out what doesn't.

Decide on a time to work on your body and healing every day, and decide what changes you will make every day to have a healthier lifestyle. This may mean turning off the TV and reading a good book. This may mean turning off the radio in your car and focusing on the sensations coming from your scar as you work with it while driving. (But be a safe driver, because that's also a part of a healthy lifestyle.)

I mentioned that your goal should be SMART.

 Why did you capitalize all of the letters in SMART?

Because SMART is an acronym. It stands for Strategic, Manageable, Attainable, Realistic, and Tangible. If your goal meets these criteria, and if you've honestly put together what you feel is a solid plan, then meet with someone whom you trust, and whose opinion on health and wellness you respect, and let them be sure you're right.

Having SMART goals with regard to your healing will help you begin with the end in mind. It doesn't mean that your plans and goals won't change as you go through the process, but here is the hazard of not beginning with the end in mind.

If you do not plan in advance, and begin with the end in mind, you can end up spending hours of time not doing the proper activities to do your healing.

So put together a plan, and know WHY that plan is there Put it someplace you can see it every day, and remind yourself why you're willing to take the time you need. What will it mean when you can move your arm like you used to? What will it mean when the scar tissue goes back to being relatively normal skin with normal sensations? Know WHY you're willing to do the healing. If you don't, then you risk letting life get in the way and you risk not taking the time you need to heal.

#3. 15 per day

Healing is a long-term process. So unlike a project where there is a clear start and finish, your healing will be ongoing. However, you need to have some tangible results, right? These tangible results are what will keep you encouraged and motivated.

So, to be realistic, I'm going to give you this expectation right up front. Working on your healing for at least 15 minutes/day, it probably will take 6 months to get to where you are starting to see some results. Just like going to the gym doesn't typically bring instant results, neither does healing. However, if you can break down the larger healing into 15 minute sessions, you will generally be more satisfied with your results. Now, there will absolutely be days when you do not want to do your 15 minutes/day, but those are the days when you especially need to. Make it a point, every day, whether it's in your car, or in front of the TV, or while you're on the phone, to do some conscious healing. (Of course it's best if you can just devote a solid 15 minutes, but if you can't, then take 5 minutes here and 5 minutes there. Use your pockets!) It will work, and you can do it!

#4. Bring it all together

In month 5, if you've truly done 15 minutes/day, you will realize how valuable your pockets really are, because you've taken 15 minutes/day and started to see some tangible results. You will feel like you can move easier, you will have reduced the appearance of the scar tissue, you will have more energy later on in the day as you do some stretching every day, etc. You will have done it all in the pockets of time you have.

#5. Continue the process

In month 6, you may want to evaluate what kind of a plan you want to put together for the healing you'll do for the **next** six months. Is 15 minutes/day enough? Would it be better to bump that time to 20 minutes/day? Evaluate how you spend your 15 minutes every day. (What kinds of activities are you doing? Might you be able to expand into doing some new kinds of activities? Are the activities you're currently doing promoting enough healing in your body? Only you can answer this question accurately, but, as always, have someone else review your plan to see if they might be able to help you think of some things you haven't thought of already.)

Use the pockets of time you have, and instead of (or at least in addition to,) watching someone else on TV get the body they want, have an instant healing, have an instant "extreme makeover," or some other such story, start healing through your own daily activities. You can do it if you realize that you do have small pockets of time, and then use the time in your pockets. If you're willing to do the work to make it happen, and are disciplined enough to stretch, massage (and do the other activities that work to heal your body), and you do these activities every day no matter what, then you will be successful. Start making your pockets more valuable!!!

In summary:

Work with the scar as often as you think about it.

It is possible to overwork an area, but it is not likely that you will with scar tissue.

Aim to work at a level that is uncomfortable, but not painful. It's a fine line to find, but when you find it, it is where the most growth happens.

We haven't touched on the use of hot and cold therapy very much, because it is generally better to let an experienced practitioner work on you with hot and cold therapy. Also, I don't talk about it much in the book because hot and cold therapy tend to be relatively specific to an area. However, a few notes on hot and cold therapy are included here at the end of the book for your consideration.

You usually use heat to bring blood to an area, and cold to take blood away from an area. Cold decreases swelling, while heat loosens muscles by bringing more blood into an area.

Generally speaking, you will want to take the blood away from an area before you work with scar tissue, so that it will hurt less to work with it (the cold of ice will also numb the nerves so you can work with the scar tissue). You will then want to work with the tissue that is deeper in the muscle, using cross-fibering, while it is cold.

Note: You don't want to use the point/prick method after icing an area, because cold therapy will diminish the receptor abilities of any nerves in the area.

When you are done, you will want to heat the area to bring blood in and carry away the toxins, which are released as you break up the scar tissue and open up the area. (Too much time with the heat can cause an abundance of blood in an area, which can cause swelling and a different kind of pain. Generally, 20-25 minutes with heat is a safe bet.) You will want to use moist heat if possible (i.e. a wet washcloth warmed up in the microwave or something comparable), as it will draw more fluids to the area and encourage the muscle to return to its natural state. (Don't get the heat so hot that it burns you.)

That's about all I will say about hot and cold therapy in the book. But ask your doctor, massage therapist, or chiropractor how hot and cold therapy might help you, and then compare what they say to what I've presented here.

Working with your scar tissue may hurt initially. The pain should decrease over time, but may not fully go away. Be prepared for this, but don't psyche yourself out. It does get better.

You can do the work yourself

You can have great results just from working on the scar tissue yourself. You will be most successful if you will work on it yourself because you are the only one who is with you 24 hours a day, so you can be there all the time, to have awareness about what is going on and to work on your own body's physical, mental, and emotional responses.

Even though you can and need to do the work yourself, having someone else work on you is perfectly acceptable as well. Just like it feels better to get a massage from someone else than it does to give yourself one, you may experience positive results from someone else working on you. Just make sure that you communicate with them (and that they are willing to listen) when there is too much pain, or not enough pressure, etc. Also, there may be cases where you can not reach the scar tissue (e.g. back surgery). If this is the case, have someone else work with you, and get into a regular stretching program). *Caveat: Make sure you say thank you to the person who is helping take care of you. They're much more likely to help again.*

Be patient.

The human body is an amazing city, going all day, and all night. What the body can do, if given the time and/or resources it needs, surpasses our understanding. If you re-injure the area by doing more than it can handle (e.g. bungee-jumping two weeks after surgery), don't expect your body to respond well. Also, eating well can have a huge impact on how quickly the body will heal. With regard to scar tissue, nutrition plays an important role in how quickly the body will be able to develop feeling in an area and breakdown the scar tissue. It needs the vitamins and minerals to build tissue, create chemical connections, and carry away toxins. Make sure you give your body what it needs dietetically.

Most importantly, remember that healing is as much a state of mind as anything else.

BE
then DO
then HAVE.

Too often, our western tradition of medical science encourages us to 'pop a pill' or 'cut it out.' That is not to say that Western medicine isn't excellent, and most times when Western remedies are used, they are effective. Western medicine and remedies are very often necessary. Speaking from personal experience, I know that the techniques used to repair my tendon in my finger, remove my appendix, patch my hernia, and rebuild my ACL, were all western techniques, and were all very effective and necessary (and appreciated)!

However, western medicine rarely incorporates the fact that the body has 100% of the chemicals and materials it needs to heal. If those chemicals and materials are directed properly, the body can be much more effective and efficient in doing its own healing.

Be healthy in your mind and in your philosophies. Choose, every day, to heal. This choice, more than anything else you can do, sends out some kind of vibration into the world.

It may be hard for you to believe, or maybe not, but MAKING A CHOICE to improve, and heal, every day, will actually attract contact with the kinds of information you need.

If you accept this information when it contacts you, it will get you to the proper therapies, activities, and actions. This choice will help you to do these small daily activities, every day, until you achieve the results that you expect.

Many of the small daily activities you can do are detailed in this book. I hope you will use them, and even if it's only five minutes a day, I hope you will use them every day. Try doing these activities for 15 minutes/day for 1 year. Then report back to me on your results!

Make sure you focus around the point/prick method if your scar has odd or "zingy" nerve sensations, and make sure you use cross-fibering if the scar tissue is in the muscle.

Begin with the philosophy. Believe that your scar tissue can go away.

Then take action to do the healing, and over time, you will have the healing that you expect.

Now stop monkeying around and go focus on healing!

Sources (text and pictures):

(1) http://www.webster.com
(2) http://www.brittanica.com
(3) http://www.rcsb.org/pdb/molecules/pdb4_1.html
(4) http://www.biospecifics.com/collagendefined.html
(5) http://education.vetmed.vt.edu/Curriculum/VM8054/Labs/Lab5/Examples/exfibro.htm
(6) http://www.pathcurve.com/Youthbloom/scar_removal.htm
(7) http://www.biology.eku.edu/RITCHISO/301notes3.htm
(8) http://www.caringmedical.com/symptoms/condition.asp?condition_id=1060
(9) http://www.medicalmultimediagroup.com/pated/shoulder_problems/unstableold.html
(10) www.healthcentral.com/mhc/img/img1948.cfm
(11) http://www.midwiferytoday.com/articles/uterinemassage.asp
(12) http://travel.howstuffworks.com/sunscreen1.htm
(13) http://www.calgaryarea.com/panthersportsmedicine/articles/sportstipspatellofemoral.htm
(14) http://itsb.ucsf.edu/~vcr/Evil.html
(15) http://www.straightdope.com/classics/a1_081.html
(16) http://training.seer.cancer.gov/ss_module01_breast/unit02_sec03_lymph_nodes.html
(17) http://www.prolonews.com/prolotherapy_e-newsletters_cortisone_shots.htm
(18) http://my.webmd.com/hw/health_guide_atoz/ta4743.asp

Other sources (concepts and pictures):
http://cellbio.utmb.edu/cellbio/rer1.htm
http://kidshealth.org/parent/general/body_basics/skin_hair_nails.html
http://www.ibismedical.com/healing_.html
http://www.deeptissue.com
http://www.ma.hw.ac.uk/~simonm/
http://www.willmot.com/knees/knees.html
http://ga.essortment.com/selfmassagetec_rspq.htm
http://www.holistic-online.com/massage/mas_face.htm
http://vtvt.essortment.com/howtogivefoot_rjwx.htm
http://www.bonecorrectivemassage.com/stomach.htm
http://www.thebreastsite.com/womens-health/breast-massage.aspx
http://www.bodymechanics.net/subpages/breast.htm
http://travel.howstuffworks.com/sunscreen1.htm
http://www.massagemag.com - Huge help for massage techniques for specific parts of the body.
http://www.jr2.ox.ac.uk/bandolier/booth/alternat/AT046.html
http://www.spacourse.com/effleurage__stroking_.html
http://www.stronghealth.com
www.kidshealth.org
http://www.mystic-mouse.co.uk

http://www.gemstate.net/susan/indexPSM.htm
www.spirithelps.com/remedies.htm
http://www.ayurveda.com/online%20resource/tongue_analysis.htm
http://healing.about.com/od/chakrameditate/a/chakrabath_2.htm
http://www.chakracolourtherapy.com/1317/info.php?p=5&pno=0
Carrie www.carriesclassics.com
Jason www.totalproductivitysolutions.com
http://www.wholesalemassagechairs.com/benefits-of-chair-massage.html
http://www.ancientway.com/Pages/Massage.html
http://www.babycentre.co.uk/general/3835.html
New Choices in Natural Healing, edited by Bill Gottlieb. Rodale Press, Prevention Magazine Health Books, 1995)
http://www.aromacaring.co.uk/Hand%20massage.htm

For more information on using uterine massage to help with infertility, contact the sources mentioned in this book or contact:
Larry Wurm
Clear Passage Therapies
4400 NW 23rd Ave
Gainesville, Florida 32606; Tel: 352-336-1433.
www.clearpassage.com cptherapy@aol.com.

Pictures:

- http://www.wit.ie/amt/cdoran/Home.htm
- http://www.medisave.co.uk/images/poster-Muscular-System.jpg
- http://www.mad-cow.org/collagen.gif
- http://itsb.ucsf.edu/~vcr/
- http://education.vetmed.vt.edu/Curriculum/VM8054/Labs/Lab5/Examples/_exfibro.htm
- http://www.genufix.com/acl_photos.htm
- http://www.pathcurve.com/Youthbloom/scar_removal.htm
- http://www.orthogastonia.com/patient_ed/images/elbow_fusion/elbow_fusion_surgery02.jpg
- http://www.caringmedical.com/cyberclinic/imgs/fig22-1.jpg
- http://www.ourreallybigadventure.com/southeastasia/Thailand/surgery.html
- http://dermatlas.med.jhmi.edu/derm/display.cfm?ImageID=-1920113364
- http://www.plasticsurgeonnewyork.com/pages/images/Scarrev$_1.jpg
- http://www.permanentmkup.com/belly%20scar%20healed.jpg
- http://www.medicalmultimediagroup.com/pated/shoulder_problems/unstableold.html
- www.woodhavenlabs.com/_ankle.html
- http://www.nebraskamed.com/heart/min_invasive_heart_valve_incision.cfm
- http://www.scoliosislife.net/pics/scar10-1.jpg
- http://yalenewhavenhealth.org/hwdb/images/hwstd/medical/orthoped/nr551501.jpg
- http://training.seer.cancer.gov/ss_module01_breast/unit02_sec01_anatomy.html

Massage Therapy
Safety - Precautions/ Contra-Indications

More Legal Schtuff, but also very important information

**Used with permission from
http://www.holistic-online.com/massage/mas_precautions.htm**

Certain medical conditions require the exercise of caution concerning the advisability of giving or receiving massage. If you are in any doubt, or if you are under medical supervision, check with your doctor or other qualified medical practitioner before embarking on massage therapy. This advice applies particularly in the case of cardiovascular conditions and heart disease, especially in cases of thrombosis, phlebitis, and edema.

Never massage directly over infected skin, for example where there are warts, herpes, or boils, or where there is inflammation, unexplained lumps, bruises and open cuts. While giving a massage, cover up any open cuts or scratches on your hands with a plaster or other dressing. Massage on the abdomen is best avoided during the first three months of pregnancy when the risk of miscarriage is highest.

The causes of acute back pain should first be diagnosed by a physician before receiving massage treatment. Consult a qualified medical practitioner in cases of raised temperature, infections, or contagious disease.

Seek medical advice before having a massage if you suffer from phlebitis, thrombosis, varicose veins, severe acute back pain, or fever.

Swellings, fractures, skin infections, or bruises should not be massaged. Lumps and swellings should be checked by your doctor.

Massage of the abdomen, legs, and feet should not be given during the first three months of pregnancy.

Cancer patients are best treated by specially trained practitioners who know which areas to avoid and which kind of massage is appropriate.

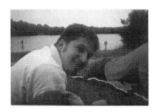

Why did I write this book?

I originally wrote an article about how to massage scar tissue and posted it on my web site. I discovered that I was getting about 3-5 emails and 1-2 phone calls every week from people who had read the article.

The article was getting over 100 visitors EVERY week!

The people who were calling and emailing were asking specific questions about how to massage specific parts of their body, how to break down scar tissue from certain kinds of trauma, and how to get more specific help. They were asking me for referrals and information, and even though I want to help everyone, it was more than I could do.

I tried to find a book to share with people, that would allow them to take their healing into their own hands, and although there are some books out about self-healing, there really isn't a good book that addresses how to work with and deal with scar tissue.

So I began writing Hey, Don't Touch Me! How to Work With Your Own Scar Tissue to Get Rid of It!

Since writing "Hey, Don't Touch Me!", I have received a lot of positive comments from people who have really been able to use the information and start to see results with their own healing. Some of those comments are posted on the next pages.

If you would like to learn more about me, it's best to visit my web site at http://www.strive4impact.com

Thank you.
The information provided is really helpful. I've been looking for some info on self healing.

Continued success to you. Take care.
Mike

Dear Mr. Kraft (Jonathan):

My husband, Greg recently tore ligaments in his right index finger and has been recovering over the past 7 weeks. Today, the hand surgeon told him that complete healing may take several months with ligament damage and that scar tissue has formed in the healing ligaments so he needs to begin strengthening the ligaments with ball squeezing and light weight movement. Anyway, Greg searched the internet for a description of and suggestions for addressing scar tissue, and he came across your informative book on the Strive 4 Impact website. One thing Greg noted to me was your emphasis on the importance of good nutrition in healing and re-creating sensation in the affected area. You seem to very much understand the role of good nutrition in health and healing. Thank-you for providing this information!

Therese

     While browsing the Internet on scar tissue - I came up with your sight. I've been searching for a few months and this was the first time I saw your sight. All others on scar tissue just say the inability to bend the knee - which I can to some degree. I had knee replacement 8 months ago and I can still feel the implant. The surgeon said that everything is fine and is it probably scar tissue. He said other than moving the knee - (he didn't give any more specific exercises) - there was nothing to be done. I was so upset when he said this. He is a top doctor in my area in computer surgery and was shocked that there is nothing he can do. I made copies of your sight and will reread. At least I know there is some hope with

massage therapy which I was never told to do. I also had that CPM machine and used it every day in rehab - but I wasn't given it to come home. I did Rehab, PT (as much as insurance would allow) and exercised at home. I don't do much now but ride the bike a little. Walking hurts my hip (which he said was probably caused from my back??)
Hate to bore you - had to vent - thanks and I'll try to follow up on your suggestions.
JZS

Dear Jonathan,
I tore a muscle when I was in Jr. High when my coach was introducing me to weight training. Doing bench presses, he added weights with each pump. I felt something pop in my right shoulder and I had to have the spotter take the bar bell away before I dropped it. It hurt initially but I had not used that muscle much so I don't notice it much. Once in a while when doing push ups or lifting above my head. More recently I have been working with weight more and I have started to notice a tightness and pain in my shoulder. It makes it difficult to do minor work using those muscles only. A while back I had heard my dad mention scar tissue in muscle injury and that prompted me to find your site. I have read your book and I agree with the physiology of it and the nature of scar tissue. I will massage my shoulder and try to (if anything) loosen up the tendons as well as stretch, as that is when it has the most sensation...I have increased my range of motion. So thank you for writing "Hey, Don't Touch Me!", it was very informative.

John W.

I recently had a world class allergic reaction in my face which apparently went into overdrive and rapidly and almost overnight formed masses of scar tissue in my cheeks, chin, lips and the side of my face. Apparently my body reacted against itself or tried to isolate something in my tissue by walling it off. In just a week, I have dense deep scar tissue causing facial deformities and surface scar tissue resembling burns.

I now have hope after reading your book. When stuff like this happens you tend to think a permanent end to it all. Your words just may prevent me from going back to that dark place. If there is anything else I can do please pass it along. I am going to recover. I look like the offspring of Andre the Giant and the Elephant man at the moment so have a long way to go.

Thank you so much, R. E.

---

thnk you for you inf,this year was my second morton neurom surgery on my right foot .(pinched nerves)i will be useing your advise..
gerald evans Orange,
US

I AM A 49YR.OLD FEMALE RUNNER THAT HAS SCAR TISSUE IN MY HAMSTRINGS AND BOTH GLUTEAL MUSCLES. I WAS VERY HAPPY TO FIND YOUR SITE. I THOUGHT I HAD RUN MY LAST MARATHON.YOUR INFO HAS GIVEN ME HOPE. I HAVE HAD MY HUSBAND MASSAGING ME ALSO USING ICE/HEAT AND STRETCHING. NOW I KNOW TO USE ICE FIRST THEN HEAT.THANK YOU AND GOD BLESS YOU. HAPPY RECOVERING RUNNER!!!!

NIRORUN

More testimonials coming soon!

Recommended Reading for BEing the kind of person who heals more easily:

Anatomy of the Spirit	Molecules of Emotion
The Way of the Peaceful Warrior	Think and Grow Rich
A Course in Miracles	How to Win Friends and Influence People
Science and Health With Key to the Scriptures	

You can also study healers throughout history
Read about stories of Jesus healing people in the Bible.
Regardless of your take on religion, Jesus is an awesome example of a healer.
Learn about St. Francis of Assisi or Padre Pio. Read about healers and you will learn what they have to teach you about healing - yourself first, then others.

Concluding thoughts

In conclusion (you cute little monkey you), there are a few things I would like to say.

First, thank-you! Your purchase of my book "How To Heal Scar Tissue" supports future research and writing I will be doing.

I really appreciate you taking the time to carefully consider purchasing this book.

I also appreciate your purchasing it!

Finally, I appreciate that you have read it through to the end. Thank-you!

Hmmm... I suppose you might have just skipped right to this page. If you did skip right to this page, then you're probably wondering, "Did I just read 'you cute little monkey you' in a book about scar tissue healing?

If that's the case, and this is the first page you have read in the entire book, then go back, and READ THE BOOK!!!

(Imagine that, someone skipping to the end of the book ... shame on you.)

And, come to think of it, yes. I did call you a monkey! Please don't eat me!

Made in United States
North Haven, CT
20 April 2025